Cardiac Surgery Procedures

Edited by Andrea Montalto, Antonio Loforte and Cristiano Amarelli

Published in London, United Kingdom

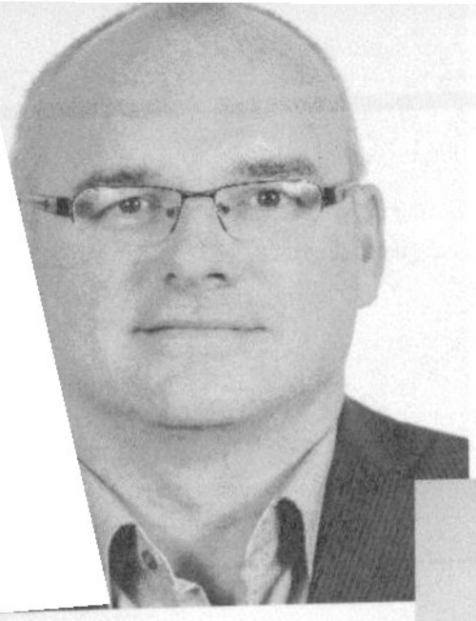
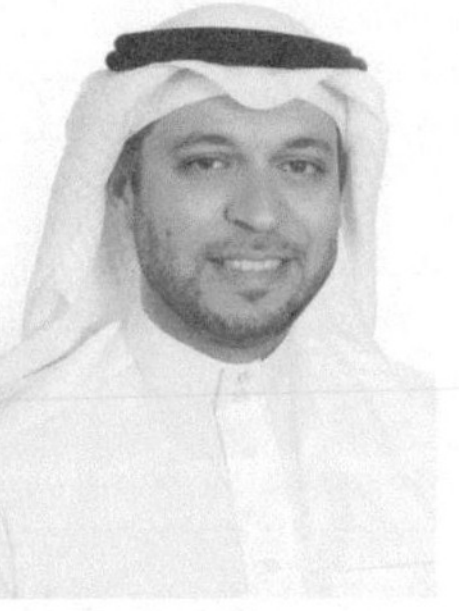
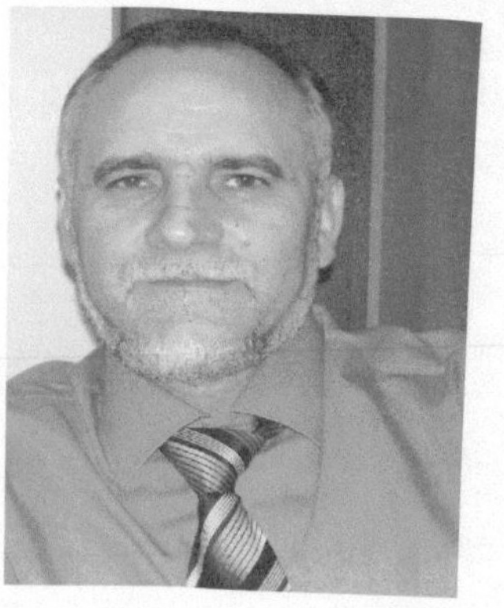
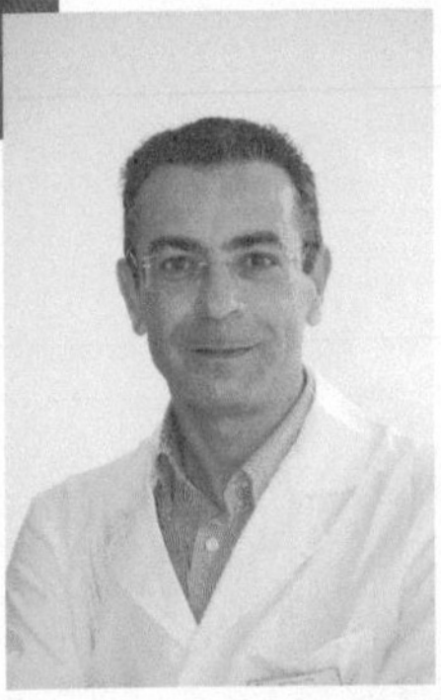
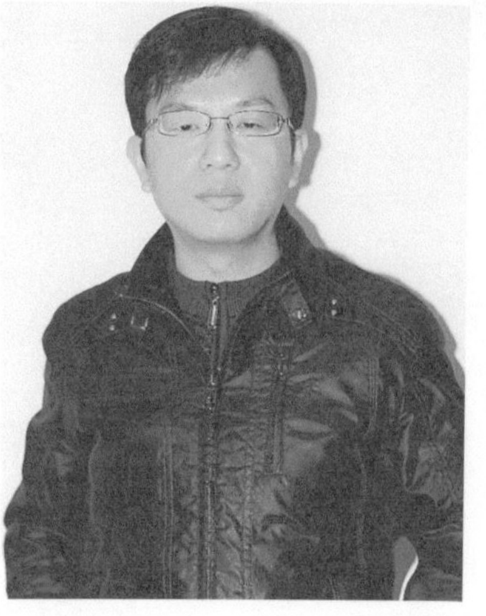
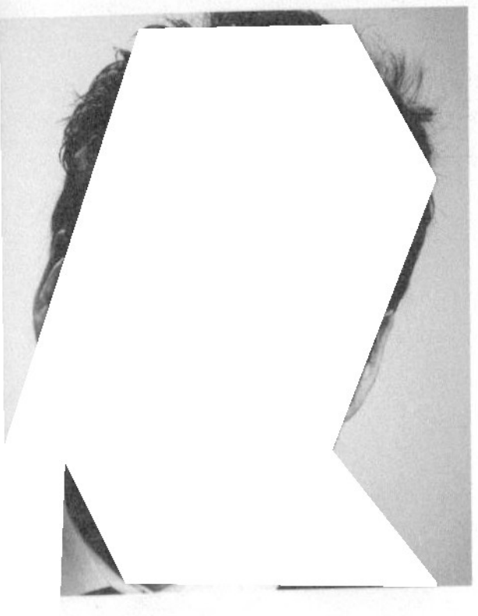
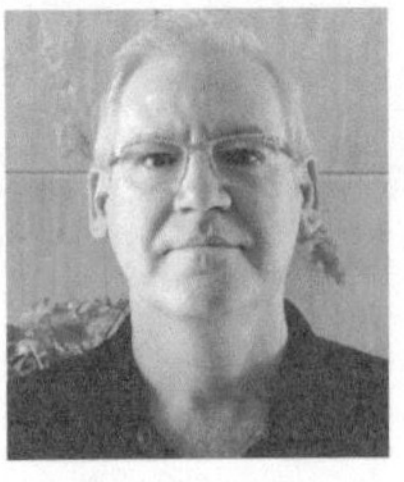

IntechOpen

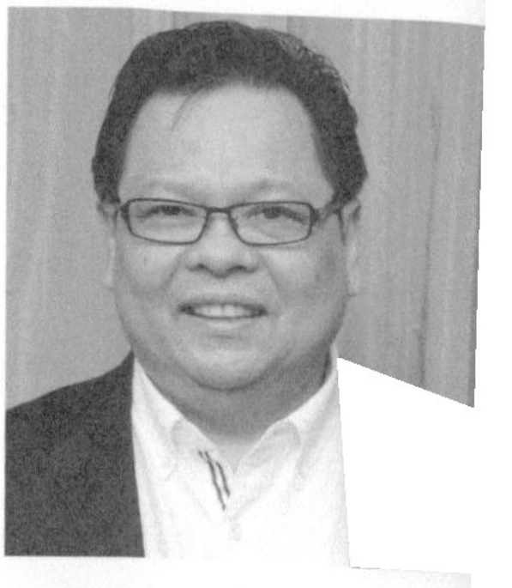
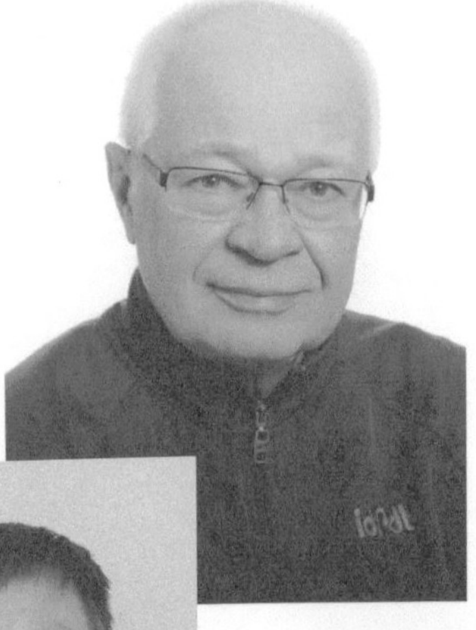
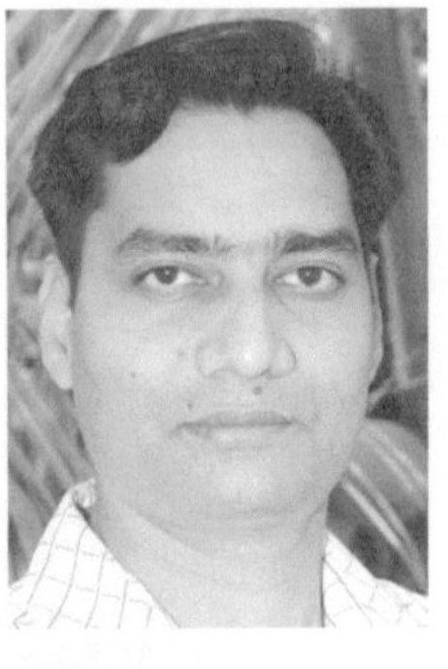
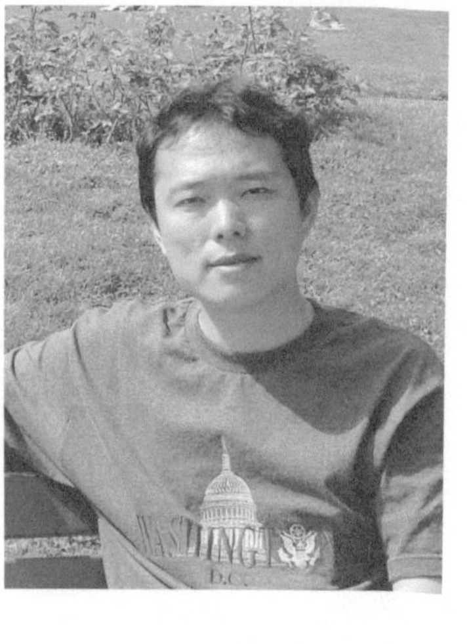
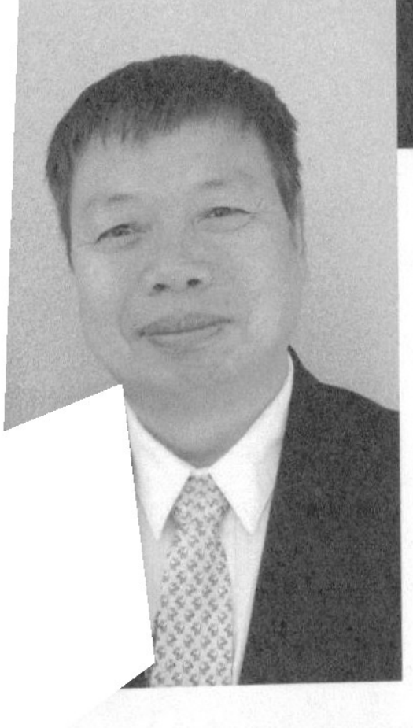
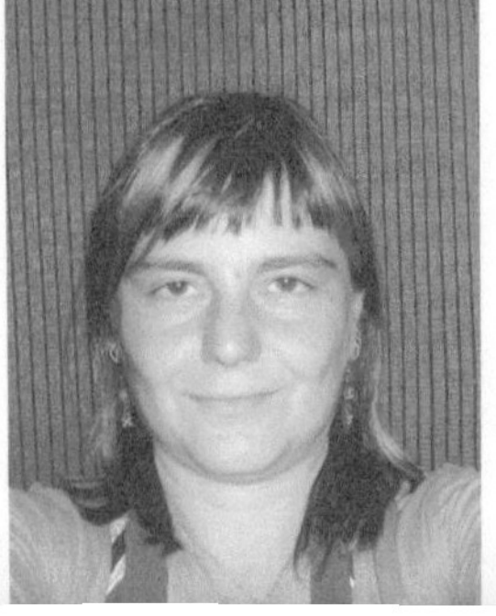

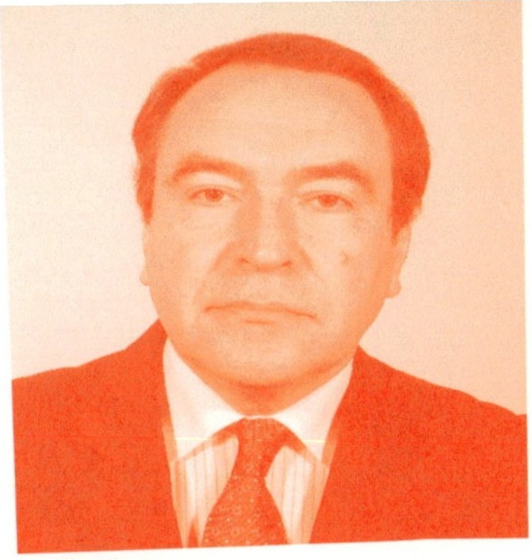
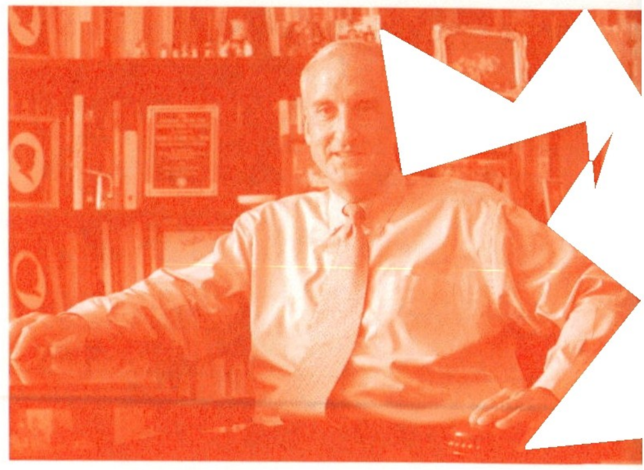
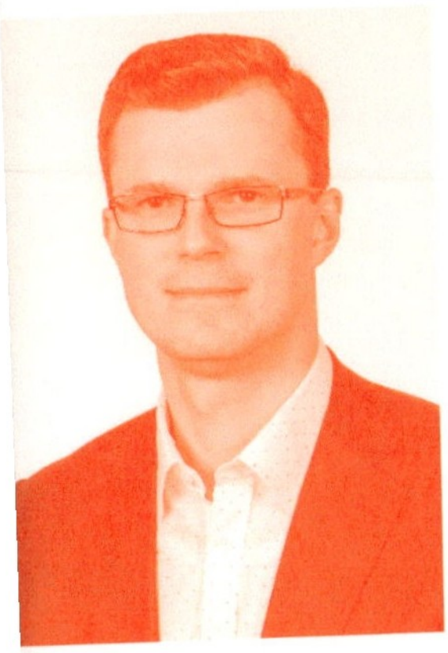
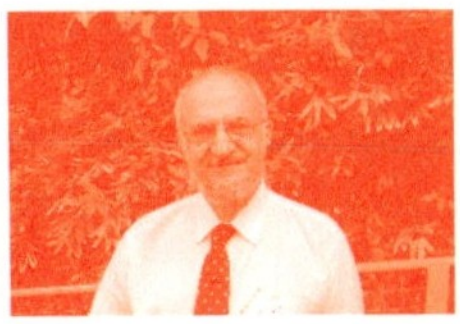
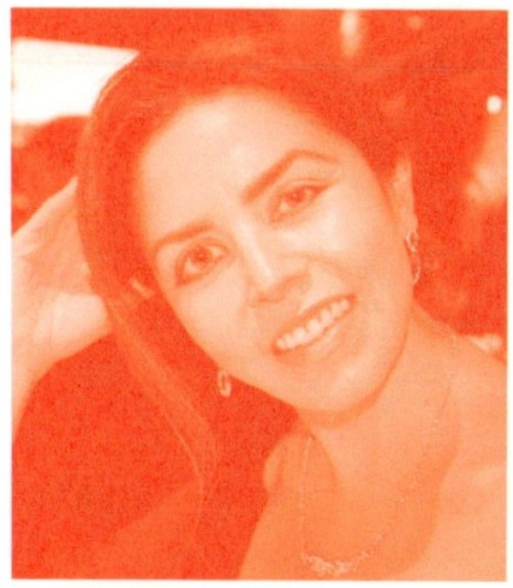

Supporting open minds since 2005

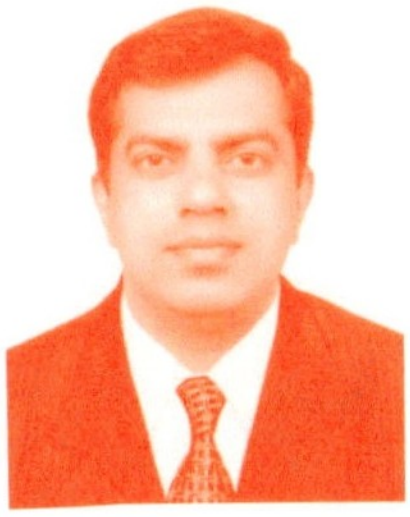
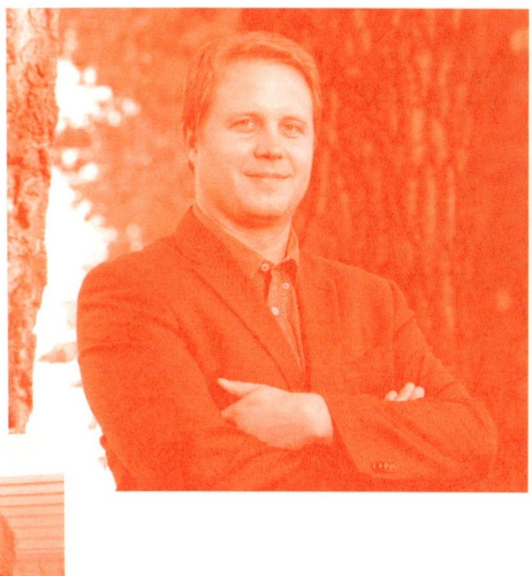
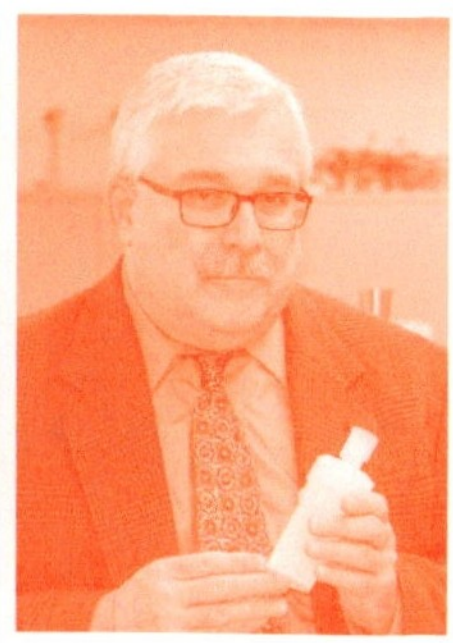
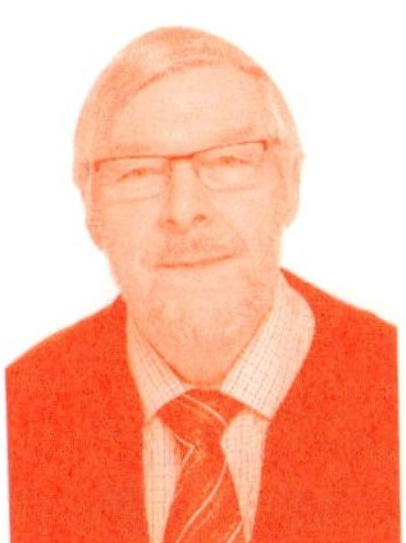
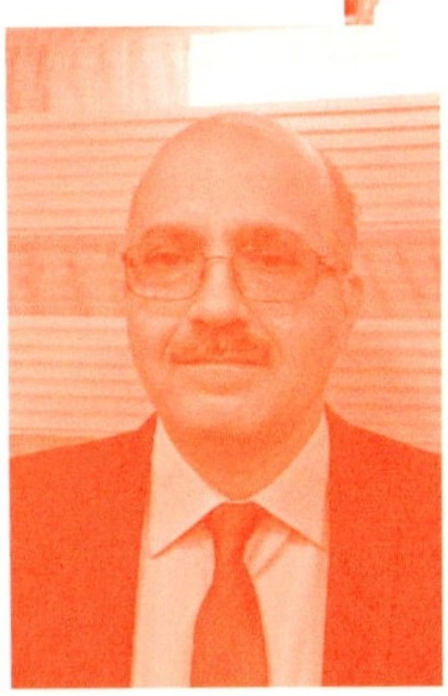
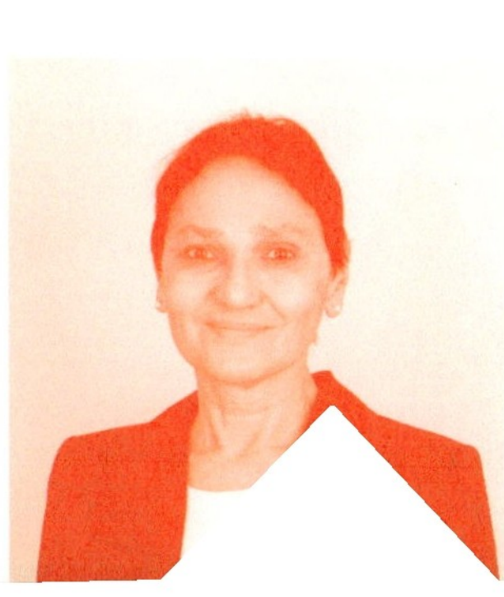
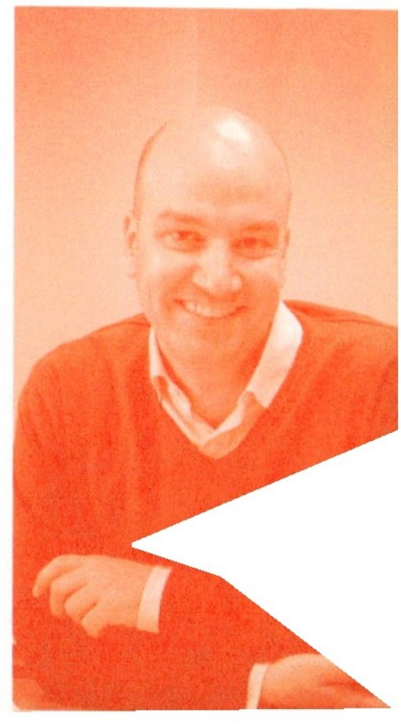

Cardiac Surgery Procedures
http://dx.doi.org/10.5772/intechopen.80835
Edited by Andrea Montalto, Antonio Loforte and Cristiano Amarelli

Contributors
Mark Slaughter, Emily Rapstine Bond, Crystal Valadon, Takashi Murashita, Yakov L Elgudin, Salil Deo, Salah Altarabsheh, Julian Smith, Imran Khan, Naresh Trehan, Massimo Antonio Padalino, Vladimiro Vida, Giovanni Stellin, Demetrio G Pittarello, Murali Prabhakaran Vettath, Kannan Arunachalam Vellachamy, Francesca Nicolò, Antonio Lio, Romina Pantanella, Roberto Scrofani, Francesco Musumeci, Marina Comisso, Antonio Giovanni Cammardella, Federico Ranocchi, Andrea Montalto, Amedeo Pergolini, Vitaliano Buffa

First published in London, United Kingdom, 2020 by IntechOpen
IntechOpen is the global imprint of INTECHOPEN LIMITED, registered in England and Wales, registration number: 11086078, 7th floor, 10 Lower Thames Street, London, EC3R 6AF, United Kingdom
Printed in Croatia

British Library Cataloguing-in-Publication Data
A catalogue record for this book is available from the British Library

Additional hard and PDF copies can be obtained from orders@intechopen.com

Cardiac Surgery Procedures
Edited by Andrea Montalto, Antonio Loforte and Cristiano Amarelli
p. cm.
Print ISBN 978-1-78984-297-5
Online ISBN 978-1-78984-298-2
eBook (PDF) ISBN 978-1-83880-272-1

For EU product safety concerns:
IN TECH d.o.o., Prolaz Marije Krucifikse Kozulić 3, 51000 Rijeka, Croatia, info@intechopen.com or visit our website at intechopen.com.

Meet the editors

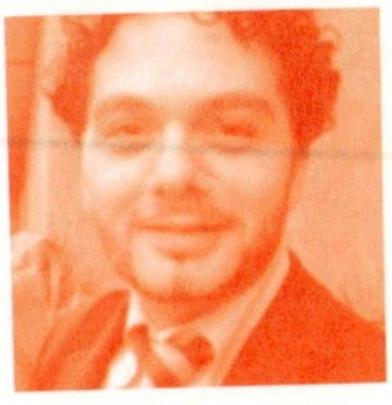

Dr. Andrea Montalto obtained his medical degree at "Federico II" University School of Medicine in Naples, Italy. After completing his residency in cardiac surgery at the University Federico II, he moved to Rome to complete his training by attending the cardiac surgery center at S. Camillo Hospital. Since 2006 he has been a permanent staff surgeon at S. Camillo Hospital, Department of Cardiac Surgery and Transplantation, Rome, Italy. Dr. Montalto has shown particular interest in the field of surgical treatment of advanced heart failure, becoming familiar in the management of patients implanted with mechanical devices. Since 2012 he has been serving as the head of the Ventricular Assist Device (VAD) program at the center of cardiac surgery at San Camillo Hospital. He is an active member of Italian Society of Cardiac Surgery (SICCH) and European Registry for Patients with Mechanical Circulatory Support (EUROMACS).

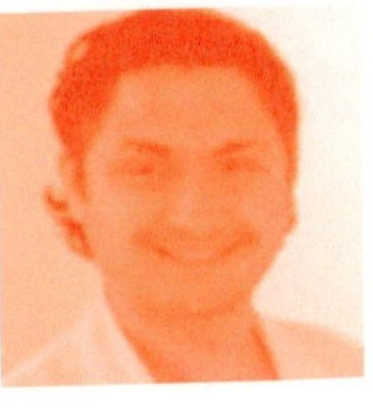

Dr. Antonio Loforte is currently a staff surgeon and co-chair of the mechanical circulatory support program at the Department of Cardiothoracic, Transplantation and Vascular Surgery, S. Orsola Hospital, Bologna University, Italy. He completed his cardiothoracic surgery residency at the University of Bologna, S. Orsola Hospital (Italy), at St. Antonius Ziekenhuis, Nieuwegein (the Netherlands), and at the Deutsches Herzzentrum, Berlin (Germany). He additionally joined the Michael E. DeBakey Department of Surgery, Division of Transplant and Assist Devices, in Houston, Texas, USA. Dr. Loforte is a member of a number of professional organizations, including the prestigious Society of Thoracic Surgeons (STS), International Society for Heart and Lung Transplantation (ISHLT), American Society for Artificial Internal Organs (ASAIO), European Association for Cardio-Thoracic Surgery (EACTS), Regional Health Improvement Collaboratives (RHICS), and Italian Society of Cardiac Surgery (SICCH) among others. His bibliography lists over 60 peer-reviewed original articles, 180 abstracts (communications) for international meetings, 10 book chapters, and one manual. He serves as a reviewer for 21 international journals and is on the editorial board of nine. He received a "European PhD label" in Organ Transplantation and three international awards in Europe and the USA.

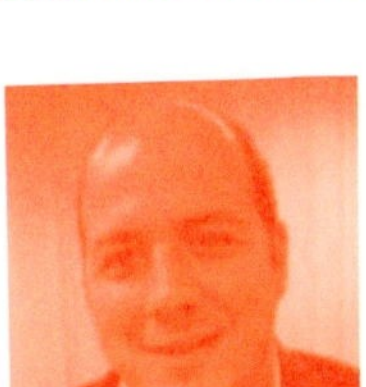

Cristiano Amarelli is a nonacademic cardiac surgeon and has been involved in the field of heart transplantation during the last 15 years with strong scientific activity in the field of transplantation, mechanical valve, and mechanical circulatory support. Born in Naples, he graduated at the Second University of Naples wherein in 2003 he completed his training in cardiovascular surgery. He is an active promoter of heart donation for the European Cardiothoracic Transplant Association (ECTTA) stimulating and coordinating the writing process of the European Consensus Conference on thoracic donors. With the European Society for Organ Transplantation (ESOT) he participates in the development of the ESOT E-learning module on transplantation whose heart module he edited with the ECTTA board. He takes an active part in the editorial board and historical committee of the American Society for Artificial Internal Organs (ASAIO) and is an active reviewer for many journals and international meetings, being named a top peer reviewer in 2017. Last year he undertook a national scheme looking to expand the adoption of mechanical circulatory support in Italy under the auspices of the National Transplant Center and the Italian Society of Cardiac Surgery. He was involved in the editorial project "Mechanical Circulatory Support in End-Stage Heart Failure."

Contents

Preface

This edited volume is a collection of reviewed and relevant research chapters, concerning developments within the cardiac surgery procedures field of study. The book includes scholarly contributions by various authors and has been edited by experts in the field. Each contribution comes as a separate chapter complete in itself but directly related to the book's topics and objectives.

The book includes chapters dealing with minimally invasive ventricular assist device surgery; cannulation for cardiopulmonary bypass; tips and pitfalls in robotic mitral valve surgery; aortic root reconstruction; minimally invasive right anterior mini-thoracotomy aortic valve replacement; minimally invasive approach in surgery for congenital heart disease; revascularization strategies in off-pump coronary artery bypass; surgical treatment of hypertrophic obstructive cardiomyopathy; and transcatheter cardiac surgery.

The target audience comprises scholars and specialists in the field.

IntechOpen

Chapter 1

Minimally Invasive Ventricular Assist Device Surgery

Marina Comisso, Andrea Montalto, Francesca Nicolò, Romina Pantanella and Francesco Musumeci

Abstract

Heart failure is a growing disease that affects millions of people around the world. Heart transplantation is currently the therapy of choice for these patients. However, the lack of donors has forced the physician to evolve another kind of therapy such as ventricular assist device (VAD) as a bridge to transplant to compensate the lack of organs. Ventricular assist devices are today a successful therapy for the treatment of heart failure; the evolution of these devices and their progressive miniaturization have allowed an evolution of their implantation technique. To date, therefore, in addition to the traditional implant through sternotomy, there are more mini-invasive implant techniques. The purpose of the treaty is to describe these techniques, the implantation sites, and the benefits they can bring to patients.

Keywords: LVAD, minimally invasive, heart failure, ventricular assist device

1. Introduction

Heart failure is a chronic progressive disease characterized by decreased pump function. This may lead to venous congestion and also to hypoperfusion due to low cardiac output with severe organ comorbidities. Modern conservative therapies for heart failure have improved outcomes in adult patients [1]. Despite medical advances in treating this condition, the disease itself remains a progressive condition. For treating end-stage heart failure, cardiac transplantation remains the gold standard. Despite this evidence, cardiac transplantation as a therapeutic option is limited by donor organ shortage and is therefore limited to patients younger than 65 years [2]. However a promising alternative to cardiac transplantation is ventricular assist device (VAD) implantation. In consideration of these problems, the number of VAD implantations has exceeded the number of cardiac transplantations [3]. This therapeutic trend, i.e., the increasing number of patients who undergo VAD implantation also as a destination therapy (DT), has led to an obvious longer duration of the assistance period with the cardiovascular assistance system. This has also led to a change in the basal characteristics of patients who (especially DT patients) are increasingly older, are more fragile, have greater comorbidities, and, consequently, may have a higher incidence of surgical complications [4]. For several years the choice approach for VAD implantation was sternotomy. However, destination therapy patients suffered a greater intraoperative risk and increased mortality [5]. Nonetheless, Slaughter showed that treatment with VADs significantly increased survival of DT patients. At that time the sternotomy approach was mandatory due to the size of the VADs [6]. Technological progress has allowed a miniaturization of the devices and their better hemodynamic performance. This has allowed the development of mini-invasive implant techniques that allow a lower surgical risk for patients, less trauma, less incidence of bleeding, and obviously less patient stay in intensive therapy [7]. The purpose of this chapter is to describe the mini-invasive VAD implantation techniques and to describe the possible benefits that these techniques can bring to the patient's outcome.

2. Indication and standard approach

The indications for the implantation of left ventricular device mainly concern patients suffering from left ventricular failure with ejection fraction ≤25% and a preserved right ventricular function (**Table 1** summarizes the main indications as indicated by the European guidelines on heart failure 2016) [8]. The standard approach for left ventricular assist device (LVAD) implantation is full sternotomy; it is done as the "first choice" in many centers around the world based on the long-term experience. The advantages of this approach are various: certainly full sternotomy provides the best anatomical overview of the heart and the major vessel and structures; moreover full sternotomy allows to approach different procedures that can be correlated and necessary to the LVAD implantation such as closure of septal defects, repair of the tricuspid valve, or ligation of the left atrium due to atrial fibrillation [9]. The classical implant operation through median sternotomy also involves the use of the heart-lung machine; the operation is divided into three main steps:

1. Connection between the left ventricle (LV) and inflow cannula.

2. Tunneling of the driveline.

3. Anastomosis of the outflow cannula to the ascending aorta.

The cannulation sites to establish the heart-lung machine are classically the right atrium and ascending aorta. The main advantages in using the heart-lung machine are two: the first one is the possibility to view and resect the trabeculae that could later cause blood turbulence and thrombus formation; the second one is the possibility to do intraoperative ventricular inspection if there's echocardiography evidence of left ventricle thrombus. However the standard surgical approach has several disadvantages: sternotomy causes pericardial adhesions and possible dangerous conditions in case of reoperations (e.g., in case of transplantation in BTT patients or in the case of pump exchange). Moreover, sternotomy leads to greater risk of postoperative bleeding, sternal infections, and wound dehiscences and therefore increases the patient's surgical trauma and risk of secondary right heart failure [7].

As previously mentioned traditionally, the implantation of the LVAD is performed with the help of the heart-lung machine. It is known, however, that this machine plays an important role in the activation of inflammatory mediators, increased pulmonary vascular resistance, platelet activation, coagulopathy, and impaired renal function [10]. The patient population that requires VAD implantation often has evidence of end-organ dysfunction, including liver congestion, renal insufficiency, and pulmonary edema. VAD placement under cardiopulmonary

Patients with severe synptoms despite optimal medical therapy and more than 1 of the following:
- LVEF < 25% and peak VO2 < 12 mL/kg/min
- ≥ 3 HF hospitalizations in previous 12 month
- Dependence on i.v. inotropic therapy
- Progressive end-organ dysfunction (worsening renal and/or hepatic function) due to reduced perfusion and not to inadequate ventricular filling pressure (PCWP ≥ 20 mmHg and C.I. ≤ 2 L/min/m²)
- Absence of severe right ventricular disfunction together with severe tricuspid regurgitation
HF, heart failure; i.v., intravenous; PCWP, pulmonary capillary wedge pressure; C.I., cardiac index.

Table 1.
Indication for implantation of LVAD.

bypass (CPB) often exacerbates these pre-existing conditions, resulting in postoperative coagulopathy, bleeding, and worsening right heart failure. VAD implantation without the use of CPB could help to minimize these postoperative complications [11].

3. Minimally invasive LVAD implantation (off-pump technique)

Minimally invasive implantation techniques require patient assessment and evaluation. Echocardiography helps identify patients with valvular disease who need concomitant valve procedure and would preferably be approached through a standard midline sternotomy. In the presence of left ventricle thrombus, an on-pump approach should be performed for thrombus removal. Noncontrast chest computed tomography is helpful in determining which intercostal space to be used and whether an anterolateral or lateral mini-thoracotomy should be utilized (most of the time, fifth or sixth intercostal space). Chest computed tomography will also be useful for the evaluation of the outflow aortic anastomosis site and to rule out aortic calcification and aneurysm [12].

The LVAD implantation is divided into three steps:

1. Inflow cannula and pump insertion.

2. Outflow graft (OG) insertion.

3. Driveline insertion.

The minimally invasive implantation procedure could be done for the first two steps.

4. Minimally invasive implantation of inflow cannula and pump insertion

There are two types of minimally invasive approaches to implant the VAD and the inflow cannula; the first one we describe is a left subcostal incision (**Figure 1**). This kind of approach was used mainly for the LVAD HeartMate II that is the largest of the contemporary LVAD devices [13]. A subcostal incision is used, running along the left-sided rib cage. After division of the abdominal muscles, preparation anteriorly to the diaphragm is performed. Through this access, the pericardium can be divided and the left ventricular apex easily identified [14].

The second one is via left anterior thoracotomy at the fifth or sixth intercostal space (**Figure 2**). Intraoperative echocardiography is used to identify the LV apex location and to determine the optimal location and intercostal space for left thoracotomy. A 6 cm thoracotomy incision is usually performed in the fifth or sixth intercostal space; upon entering the chest, the pericardium is identified and divided, and a pericardial cradle is created with pericardial sutures to expose the LV apex [12].

In case of an off-pump VAD placement, there are techniques that can be used to reduce the use of blood. Reliant on the experience in transcatheter valve implantation by the use of rapid pacing, multiple authors reported inserting off-pump LVAD with rapid pacing for the insertion [15]. Implantation of LVAD with non-fibrillatory technique by administrating of an intravenous bolus of adenosine to induce a short bradycardic arrest during off-pump LVAD placement was also described [16], in order to reduce blood loss by reducing both the volume of the blood ejected from the heart during LVAD implant (reduction in blood pressure) and decreasing the heartbeats. In this method adenosine mediates pulmonary vasodilatation, which may reduce pulmonary resistance and protect the right ventricle function [17].

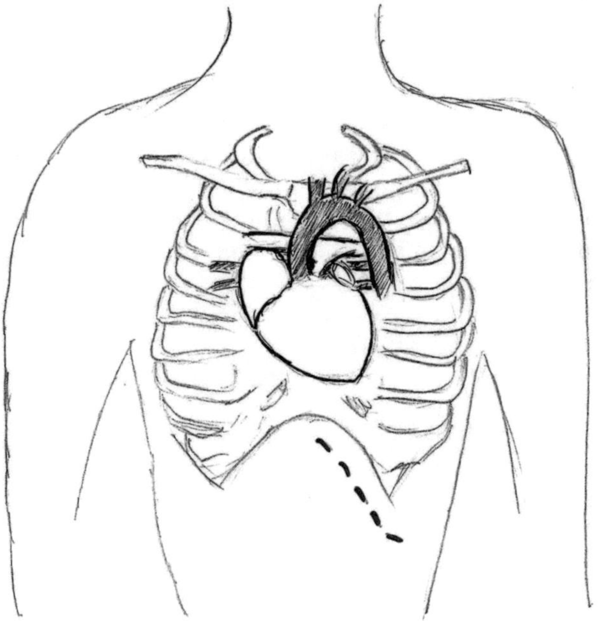

Figure 1.
Left subcostal incision.

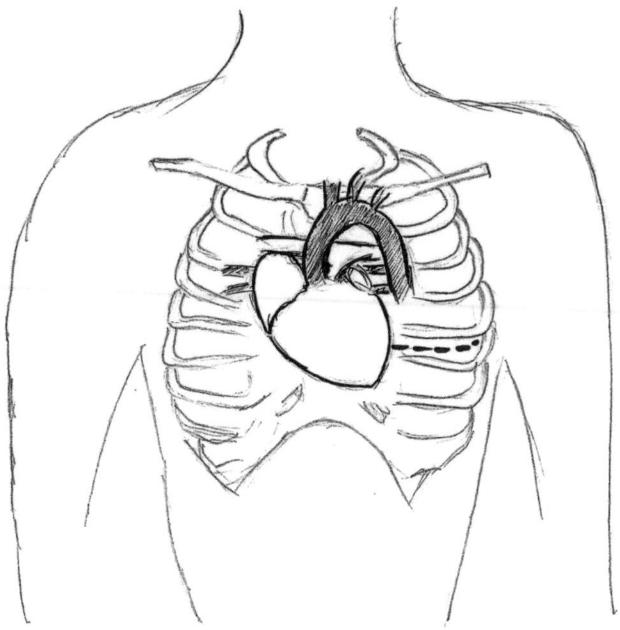

Figure 2.
Left anterior thoracotomy at fifth or sixth intercostal space.

5. Outflow graft insertion

This step of LVAD implantation technique could be done by multiple ways in different locations: right mini-thoracotomy, split upper hemi-sternotomy, axillary and subclavian arteries, supraceliac abdominal aorta, innominate artery, and descending aorta [18].

The most commonly used technique for on-pump minimally invasive strategy of LVAD implantation is through upper hemi-sternotomy (**Figure 3**) [19]. A 4 cm upper hemi-sternotomy is performed to expose the ascending aorta; if CPB is planned, the distal ascending aorta could be used for arterial cannulation to assure adequate cerebral perfusion, and femoral vein is used for a percutaneous venous cannulation. It can be associated with either inflow pump incisions; for the majority of patients, the outflow graft is tunneled and passed within the pericardium and anastomosed to the proximal ascending aorta (**Figure 4**). The OG could be passed in the anterior mediastinum behind the sternum in case of previous sternotomy.

Another way to implant the OG is through right mini-thoracotomy (**Figure 5**). This kind of approach can be used if the ascending aorta demonstrated a right-side curvature on preoperative chest tomography. A 4–6 cm incision is made at second to third intercostal spaces which allows access to the ascending aorta to perform the outflow anastomosis: after passing the outflow graft from the left thoracotomy to the right thoracotomy, a side-biting clamp is attached on the ascending aorta, and after adequate incision of the aorta, the graft is anastomosed in the usual manner. Another method is the combination of the previous two approaches through an upper hemi-sternotomy with right hemi-thoracotomy J-shape incision (**Figure 6**). At least left subclavian outflow graft anastomosis has been increasingly utilized for patient's anatomy when OG anastomosis to the ascending or the descending aorta is prohibited (**Figure 7**). The OG is tunneled through the right or the left pleural cavity and passed through the second intercostal space to be anastomosed to the subclavian artery (**Figure 8**). If this technique is used, attention must be paid to the eventual

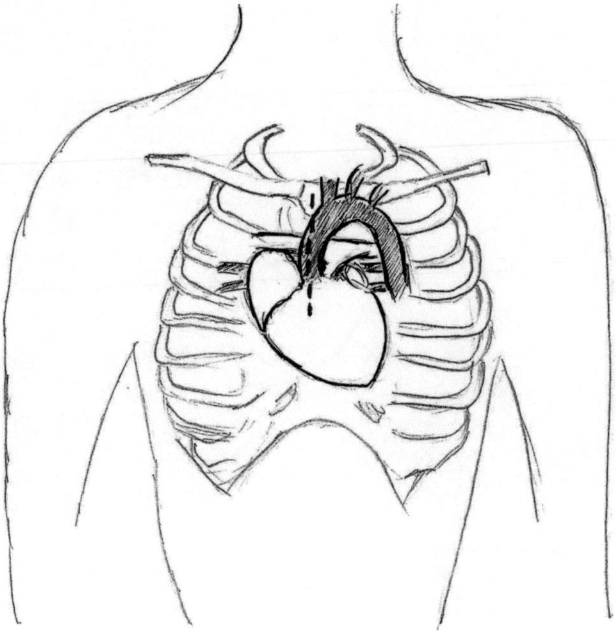

Figure 3.
Upper hemi-sternotomy.

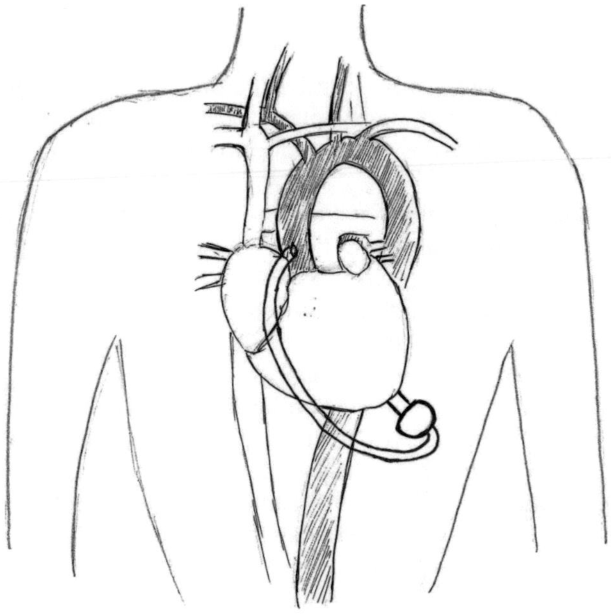

Figure 4.
The OG anastomosed to the proximal ascending aorta.

compression of the OG by adjacent structures; it is necessary to reduce the possibility of creating excess flow to the arm and also the turbulence of the flow in case of mobilization of the arm. Banding of the subclavian artery is mandatory if there is a mean pressure difference of more than 20 mmHg to avoid excessive blood flow to the arm [20].

Two further types of approaches are used less frequently: single left thoracotomy incision with descending aorta anastomosis (**Figure 9**) and supraceliac

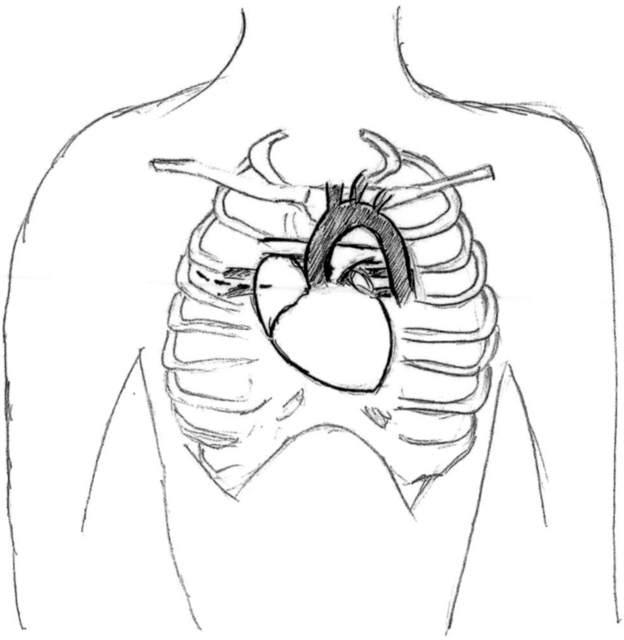

Figure 5.
Right hemi-thoracotomy.

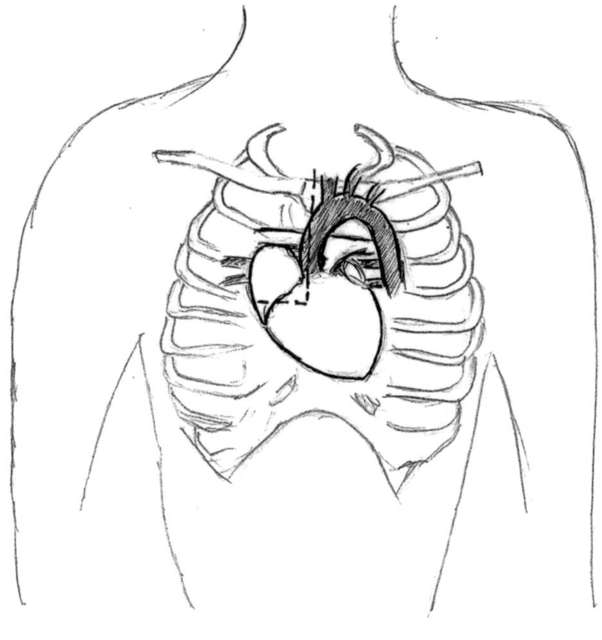

Figure 6.
Right hemi-sternotomy J-shape incision.

abdominal aorta anastomosis (**Figure 10**). In the first approach, the inferior pulmonary ligament is freed to optimize exposure; the OG is placed in the left pulmonary fissure, measured, and anastomosed end to side to the descending aorta or the aortic arch using a partial cross clamp [21]. The second one is used by making left subcostal incision and dividing the diaphragm to make the pocket. This allows the LVAD to be implanted on the diaphragmatic surface of the left ventricle, and the supraceliac aorta is then exposed by extraperitoneal exposure. The outflow is trimmed and anastomosed end to side on the supraceliac aorta [22].

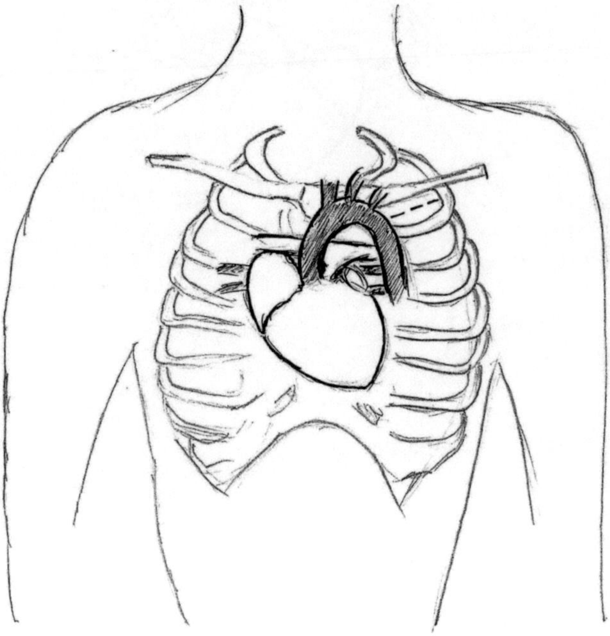

Figure 7.
Left hemi-thoracotomy.

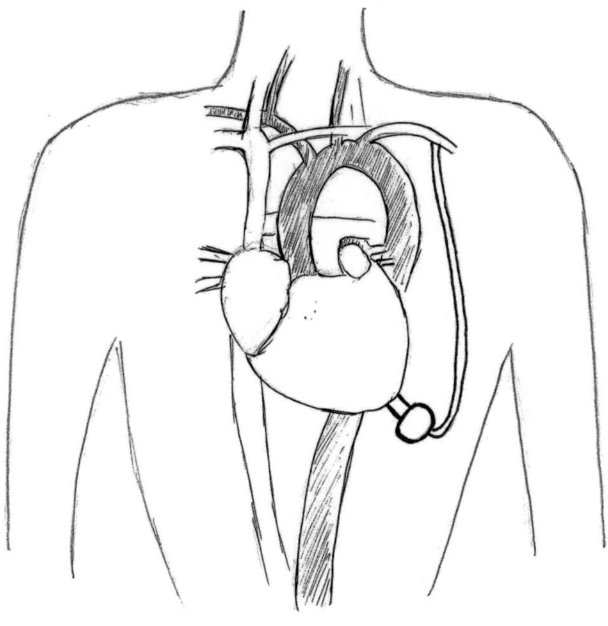

Figure 8.
The OG anastomosed to the subclavian artery.

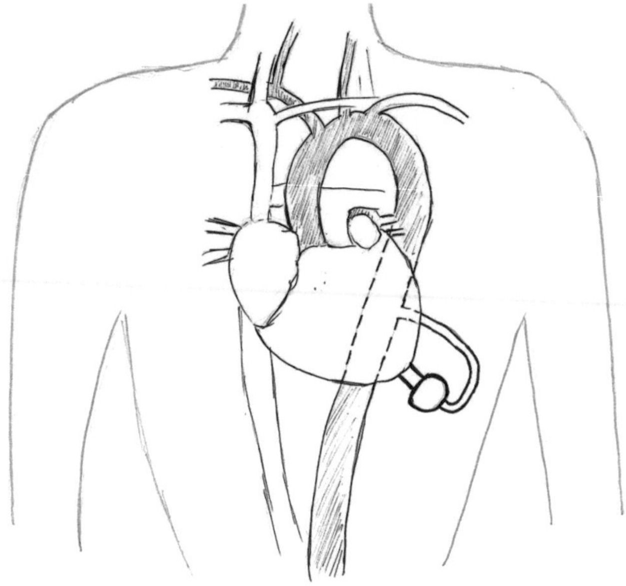

Figure 9.
Single left thoracotomy incision with descending aorta anastomosis.

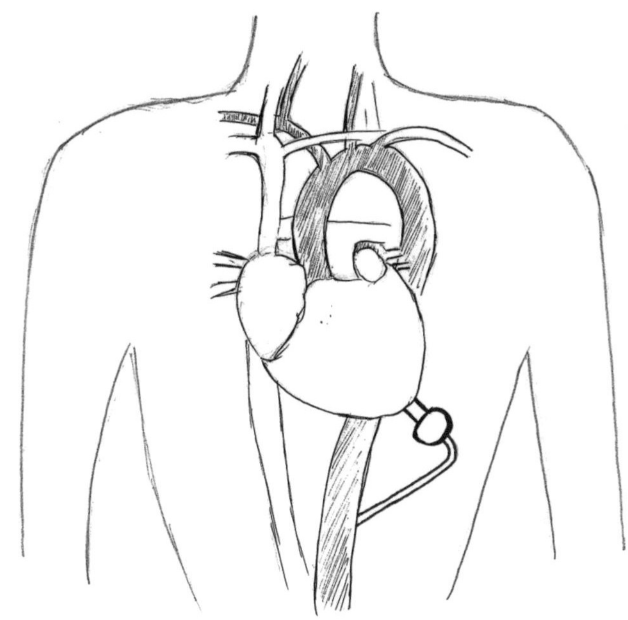

Figure 10.
Supraceliac abdominal aorta anastomosis.

6. Conclusions

The use of LVAD has increased significantly along with the rapidly expanding heart failure patient population. Like in other cardiac surgical procedures, minimally invasive approaches are becoming more commonly used, also in the field of VAD implantation. Multiple studies have shown minimally invasive cardiac surgery improves outcomes with reduced surgical trauma and complication rates, e.g., postoperative bleeding, reduced blood transfusion requirement, faster recovery rate, and decreased hospital cost. However it remains a matter of debate if these approaches offer advantages in comparison to standard full-sternotomy access in LVAD implantation procedure. An undeniable advantage of the minimally invasive implantation technique is the lack of adhesions at the time of transplant, which facilitates heart transplantation and also reduces ischemia time resulting in improved graft performance. The use of off-pump LVAD implantation approach allows the avoidance of cardiopulmonary bypass and will decrease the incidence of vasoplegia and coagulopathy postoperatively. Another advantage of a less invasive approach is that the right ventricle remains in its natural position, as the surrounding pericardium stays intact and the right ventricular function remains sustained; in this way right ventricular failure is passively avoided [23]. The progressive miniaturization of VADs has provided a further boost to the research of mini-invasive implantation techniques, and future research will tend towards ever greater device miniaturization. LVAD implantation by minimally invasive procedure is feasible and safe; LVAD implantation without the use of CPB has the potential to minimize postoperative complication such as excessive bleeding during implantation without compromising hemodynamics. By minimizing the needs for blood transfusions, patients have decreased exposure to blood antigens which ultimately reduces the risk of sensitization in BT patients. The upcoming advancement of LVAD technology and miniaturization of mechanical circulatory support will only further advance the success of LVAD surgery and will benefit more patients especially with the rapidly growing heart failure population worldwide.

Conflict of interest

The author has no conflicts of interest to declare.

Notes/Thanks/Other declarations

We would like to thank S. Castellan for her work on the figures.

Author details

Marina Comisso[1*], Andrea Montalto[1], Francesca Nicolò[1], Romina Pantanella[2] and Francesco Musumeci[1]

1 Department of Cardiac Surgery and Heart Transplantation, San Camillo Hospital, Rome, Italy

2 Department of Cardiac Surgery, Sant Andrea Hospital, Rome, Italy

*Address all correspondence to: marina.comisso@gmail.com

References

[1] Nair AP, Timoh T, Fuster V. Contemporary medical management of systolic heart failure. Circulation Journal. 2012;**76**:268-277

[2] Lund LH, Edwards LB, Kucheryavaya AY, et al. The registry of the International Society for Heart and Lung Transplantation: Thirty-second official adult heart transplantation report–2015; focus theme: Early graft failure. The Journal of Heart and Lung Transplantation. 2015;**34**:1244-1254

[3] Kirklin JK, Naftel DC, Pagani FD, et al. Seventh INTERMACS annual report: 15000 patients and counting. The Journal of Heart and Lung Transplantation. 2015;**34**:1495-1504

[4] Moazami N, Milano CA, John R, et al. Pump replacement for left ventricular assist device failure can be done safety and is associated with low mortality. The Annals of Thoracic Surgery. 2013;**95**:500-505

[5] Coyle LA, Ising MS, Gallagher C, et al. Destination therapy: One year outcome in patients with a body mass index greater than 30. Artificial Organs. 2010;**34**:93-97

[6] Slaughter MS, Rogers JG, Milano CA, et al. Advanced heart failure treated with continuous-flow left ventricular device. The New England Journal of Medicine. 3 Dec 2009;**361**(23):2241-2251

[7] Hanke JS, Rojas SV, Avsar M, et al. Minimally-invasive LVAD implantation: State of the art. Current Cardiology Reviews. 2015;**11**:246-251

[8] Ponikowski P, Voor AA, Anker SD, et al. 2016 ESC guidelines for the diagnosis and treatment of acute and chronic heart failure. European Journal of Heart Failure. 2016;**18**:891-975

[9] Balsara KR, Bierhals A, Vader J, et al. Implantation of left ventricular assist device in patient with left ventricular non-compaction. Journal of Cardiac Surgery. Feb 2017;**32**(2):159-161

[10] Belhaj A. Actual knowledge of systemic inflammation reaction during cardiopulmonary bypass. Recent Patents on Cardiovascular Drug Discovery. 2012;**7**:165-169

[11] Cheung A, Lamarche Y, Kaan A, et al. Off-pump implantation of the HeartWare HVAD left ventricular assist device through minimally invasive incision. The Annals of Thoracic Surgery. 2011;**91**:1294-1296

[12] Cheng A. Minimally invasive left ventricular assist device placement. Journal of Visceral Surgery. 2015;**1**:25

[13] Pagani FD, Miller LW, Russel SD, et al. Extended mechanical circulatory support with continuous-flow rotary left ventricular assist device. Journal of the American College of Cardiology. 2009;**54**:312-321

[14] Wiedemann D, Haberl T, et al. Minimally invasive approaches for implantation of left ventricular assist device. Indian Journal of Thoracic and Cardiovascular Surgery. 2018;**34**(Suppl 2):S177-S182

[15] Centofanti P, La Torre M, Attisani M, et al. Rapid pacing for the off-pump insertion of the Jarvik left ventricular assist device. The Annals of Thoracic Surgery. 2011;**92**:1536-1538

[16] Maltais S, Davis ME, Haglund N. Minimally invasive and alternative approaches for long term LVAD placement: The Vanderbilt strategy. Annals of Cardiothoracic Surgery. 2014;**3**:563-569

[17] Galiè N, Ussia G, Passarelli P, et al. Role of pharmacologic tests in the treatment of primary pulmonary

hypertension. The American Journal of Cardiology. 1995;**75**:55A-62A

[18] El-Sayed Ahmed MM, Aftab M, Singh SK, et al. Left ventricular assist device outflow graft: Alternative sites. Annals of Cardiothoracic Surgery. 2014;**3**(5):541-545

[19] Ricklefs M, Hanke SJ, Schmitto JD, et al. Less invasive surgical approaches for left ventricular assist device implantation. Seminars in Thoracic & Cardiovascular Surgery. 2018;**30**(1):1-6. DOI: 10.1053/j.semtcvs.2018.01.002

[20] Riebandt J, Sandner S, Mahr S, et al. Minimally invasive thoratec Heartmate II implantation in the setting of severe thoracic aortic calcification. The Annals of Thoracic Surgery. 2013;**96**:1094-1096

[21] Popov AF, Mohite PN, Sabashnikov A, et al. Minimally invasive HeartWare LVAD implantation through single left thoracotomy. Journal of Artificial Organs. 2015;**18**:170-172

[22] Anyanwu AC. Technique for less invasive implantation of HeartMate II left ventricular assist device without median sternotomy. Seminars in Thoracic and Cardiovascular Surgery. 2011 Autumn;**23**(3):241-244

[23] Schmitto JD, Molitoris U, Haverich A, et al. Implantation of a centrifugal pump as a left ventricular assist device through a novel, minimized approach: Upper hemisternotomy combined with anterolateral thoracotomy. The Journal of Thoracic and Cardiovascular Surgery. 2012;**143**:511-513

Chapter 2

Cannulation for Cardiopulmonary Bypass

Emily Bond, Crystal Valadon and Mark Slaughter

Abstract

Cardiac surgery has made significant progress since the advent of cardiopulmonary bypass. Arterial cannulation for bypass is a cornerstone to most cardiac procedures. Choosing an ideal cannulation site, employing peri- and intraoperative imaging, selecting an appropriate cannula, and avoiding complications are vital to success. These, along with the steps to arterial cannulation, are discussed in this chapter.

Keywords: cardiopulmonary bypass, arterial cannulation, aortic cannulation, femoral cannulation, axillary cannulation

1. Introduction

Cardiopulmonary bypass serves the purpose of acting in place of the patient's heart and lungs during a cardiac operative procedure. The mechanism allows for blood to become reoxygenated in order to ensure sufficient perfusion throughout the patient's body. The application of this novel concept is attributed to John Gibbon Jr., and its first successful clinical use was reported in 1953 [1]. However, it did not become more practically available until in 1955 when both John Kirklin at the Mayo Clinic and C. Walton Lillehei at the University of Minnesota introduced its routine use in open heart surgery [1].

The utilization of cardiopulmonary bypass increased significantly between the years 1960 and 1969 due to the increased demand brought on by advances in the field of cardiothoracic surgery. Prior to this era, the majority of cardiac surgeries being performed addressed congenital heart disease in an expeditious fashion. Bypass allowed more complex problems to be repaired by allowing more time for the surgeon to operate while the patient maintained perfusion. Additionally, the need for reliable extracorporeal circulation was expanded with the introduction of coronary artery bypass grafting, the development of artificial heart valves, the utilization of deep hypothermia to facilitate circulatory arrest, and heart transplantation [1].

With the use of cardiopulmonary bypass increasing so dramatically, research into further understanding and improvement of the process was initiated, particularly in the 1980s. Special investigative attention was given to the inflammatory reaction induced by cardiopulmonary bypass, the development of drugs to reduce adverse neurologic events, and flow pulsatility [1–3]. The field of cardiothoracic surgery and the advancement of cardiopulmonary bypass have continued to be refined and improved.

2. Arterial cannulation sites

Arterial cannulation is necessary in order to provide oxygenated blood systemically during cardiopulmonary bypass. Currently, there are three different sites that can be utilized to achieve this function:

- Distal ascending aorta
- Femoral artery
- Axillary artery

The most commonly utilized site is the distal ascending aorta. In this instance, cannulation is performed near the origin of the brachiocephalic trunk [4]. In the event this site is not a viable option, the femoral artery is the standard peripheral site. Femoral arterial cannulation can be accessed both by open cutdown technique and percutaneous techniques. If a percutaneous approach is taken, the arteriotomy will need to be closed using a percutaneous vessel closure device or an open repair. If both the distal ascending aorta and femoral artery prove to be high-risk options due to complications, the axillary artery is the next alternative, preferably on the right side. This vessel is accessed via the deltopectoral groove via a standard infraclavicular cutdown.

3. How to choose the appropriate arterial cannulation site

Determining which arterial cannulation site to use depends on factors such as the procedure being performed, patient body habitus, and the degree of atherosclerotic disease present [5]. Therefore, each case should be evaluated individually to decide upon the best course of action. Based on the surgical procedure, it must be determined if the distal ascending aorta is an appropriate cannulation site. Instances where this may not be the case include repeat sternotomy, emergency surgery, minimally invasive surgery, anatomic anomalies, prohibitive atherosclerotic disease, and robotic cardiac surgery, among others [4]. The benefits of antegrade versus retrograde flow must also be weighed. Both the distal ascending aorta and the axillary artery have the advantage of anterograde flow, whereas the femoral artery exhibits retrograde flow [5]. This is especially important in cases involving aortic dissection. When contemplating using femoral access, excessive arterial calcification, previous groin operations, and body habitus must be considered.

4. Preoperative imaging

Obtaining the appropriate imaging studies prior to conducting cardiopulmonary bypass is essential, as the information gathered can influence the surgical approach. There are several different imaging options that can be utilized. The most routine preoperative imaging study performed is chest radiography. Chest x-ray (anteroposterior and lateral) can provide information such as the size and shape of the cardiac silhouette, traces of previous thoracic interventions or hardware, severe atherosclerotic disease, and significant pulmonary disorders, in addition to other pertinent information [6]. In the current era, nearly every patient who presents with chest pain has CT imaging ordered by a provider during the work-up. Chest CT can provide an abundance of information regarding the patient's anatomy and quality of vasculature, as well as many anomalies and abnormalities. Certain findings such as porcelain aorta, dissections, and subclavian stenosis can alter the operative treatment plan. Recent data has suggested that CT should be the standard preoperative imaging for patients with prior sternotomy, as doing so has been associated with a lower risk of perioperative complication [7]. This type of imaging allows for the surgeon to visualize and analyze the sternum more effectively, providing information that will ultimately optimize planning of the surgical procedure [7].

Additional imaging modalities that can be utilized preoperatively include transesophageal echocardiogram (TEE) and transthoracic echocardiogram (TTE). Echocardiography has the ability to provide critical information in order to optimize hemodynamics and identify conditions that had not been appreciated on static imaging [8]. In regard to determining which form of echocardiography (TEE vs. TTE) is most appropriate, several factors should be considered. The imaging quality of TTE is limited by the structures the signal must traverse. TEE has shown to provide superior imaging, particularly for posterior structures that are closer in association to the esophagus including the aorta and both atria [9]. The disadvantages of TEE in comparison to TTE include its invasive nature, requirement for sedation, and increased time to perform. Despite these factors, TEE's improved ability to visualize critical structures suggests that it should be the echocardiography imaging of choice for procedures requiring cardiopulmonary bypass. In our practice, TEE is regularly performed in the operating room after induction and prior to incision to verify and support the other preoperative cardiac function tests.

5. Types of cannulas

Aortic cannulas come in a variety of commercially available options. Cannula size should be selected in conjunction with the perfusionist team so as to utilize the appropriate cannula for adequate flow within the circuit. Too large of a cannula may require an aortotomy that is difficult to close in a standard fashion, while too small of a cannula will not allow sufficient flows. A narrower cannula can cause high pressure gradients, cavitation, or jets of flow which can increase the likelihood of dissection. Diffusion-tip cannulas are available which provide multidirectional flow to reduce jets. The tip of the cannula may be straight, tapered, or angled, as well as made from metal or plastic. Various tip modifications, such as flanges or adjustable rings, are available to prevent the cannula from being inserted too far into the aorta and impeding flow to the head vessels. When using an alternate arterial cannulation site, certain adjustments must be made. Adequate bypass support via femoral cannulation is best achieved with a long, wire-reinforced cannula, whereas the diameter of the axillary artery must be taken into account when selecting an appropriate cannula [10].

6. Steps to cannulation

Arterial cannulation is almost always completed prior to venous cannulation during the setup for cardiopulmonary bypass. The steps below outline the appropriate manner in which arterial cannulation can be achieved.

1. Identify the appropriate cannulation site through the use of preoperative imaging, surgical history, and operator preference (**Figure 1**).

2. Utilize additional intraoperative imaging, such as TEE and epi-aortic ultrasound (discussed below), and surgical palpation to ensure avoidance of atherosclerotic regions to minimize risk of embolization. Adequate surgical exposure should be obtained through tedious dissection of the desired vessel. When using the axillary or femoral artery, proximal and distal control should be obtained in the form of vessel loops. Ascending aortic exposure should include the origin identification and isolation of the brachiocephalic trunk and the main pulmonary artery, at a minimum.

3. Two purse string sutures should be placed at the intended access site, typically with monofilament (Prolene™) or braided (Ethibond™) nonabsorbable suture, at a distance that can accommodate an average 20–22F cannula (**Figure 2**).

These should be snared in the standard fashion, as they will be tightened and tied after the cannula has been removed to close the aortotomy. The adventitia within the sutures is then gently divided to prepare for aortotomy (**Figure 3**).

4. Close attention should be paid to the systemic blood pressure, which should be below 100 mmHg prior to aortotomy to decrease the incidence of dissection. A #11 or #15 blade is used to make the aortotomy within the purse string sutures, while the adventitia superior to the incision is pulled gently inferiorly to cover the defect in order to prevent excessive bleeding (**Figure 4**). The incision should be adequate to accommodate the selected cannula but not excessively wide so as to cause difficulty snaring the cannula in place while on bypass. The selected cannula is then inserted into the aorta, and the sutures snared down (**Figure 5**). As previously mentioned, the cannula tip should not be inserted any further than necessary so as to provide optimal systemic flow.

5. Appropriate placement of the cannula is then verified by checking for adequate back-bleeding, which is an opportunity to de-air the cannula as well. Alternatively, the perfusionist may check the arterial waveform for flow verification after the line has been de-aired and connected to the circuit.

6. The arterial cannula and snares are then tied together with silk ties to provide additional stability [11] (**Figure 6**).

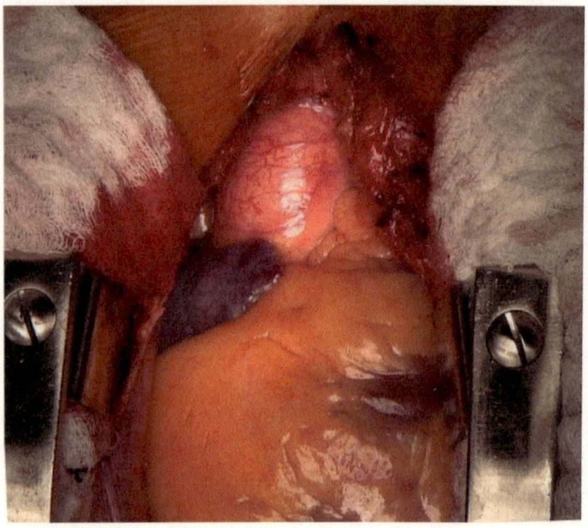

Figure 1.
Ascending aortic exposure prior to cannulation.

Closing the aortic cannulation site is rather straightforward. The purse string sutures that were placed prior to the cannula insertion are utilized to close the incision once the tubing has been removed. If needed, an additional mattress

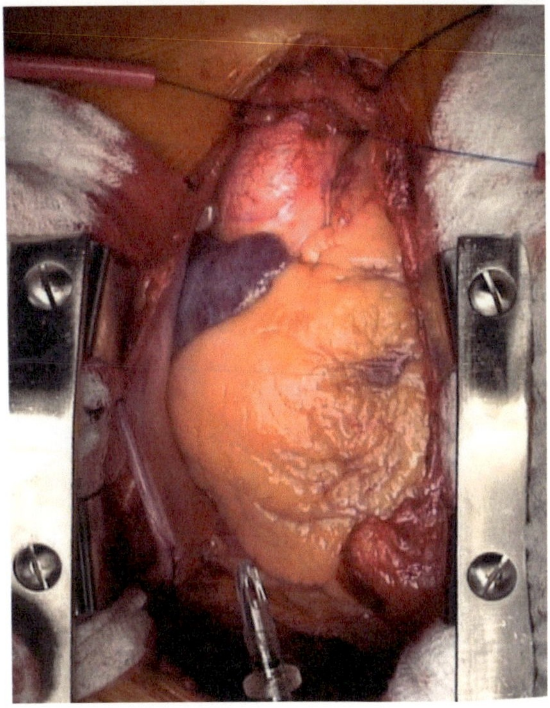

Figure 2.
Cannulation site opposite brachiocephalic artery with purse string sutures placed. Note the cannula at the lower border of the image with a flange marking the maximum length of desired insertion.

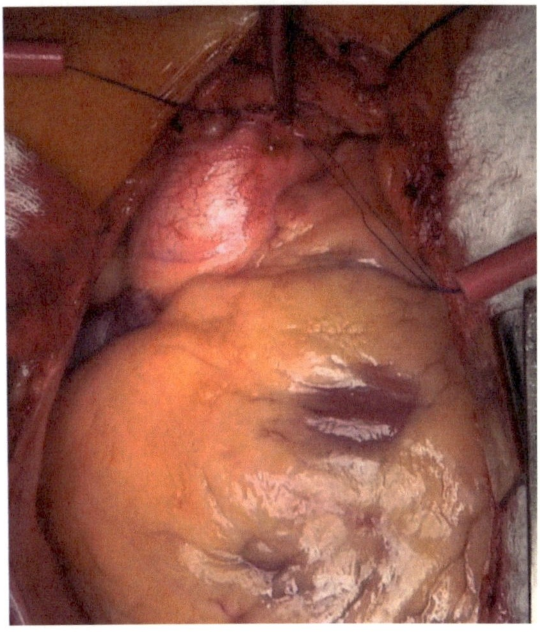

Figure 3.
The adventitia is gently removed from the cannulation site within the purse string sutures.

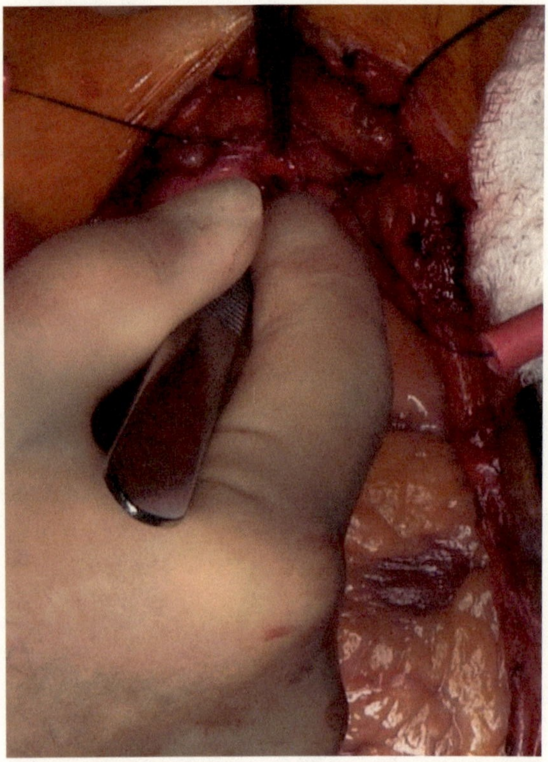

Figure 4.
A scalpel is used to make the aortotomy at the cannulation site, while gentle inferior traction is placed with the adventitia to prevent excessive bleeding.

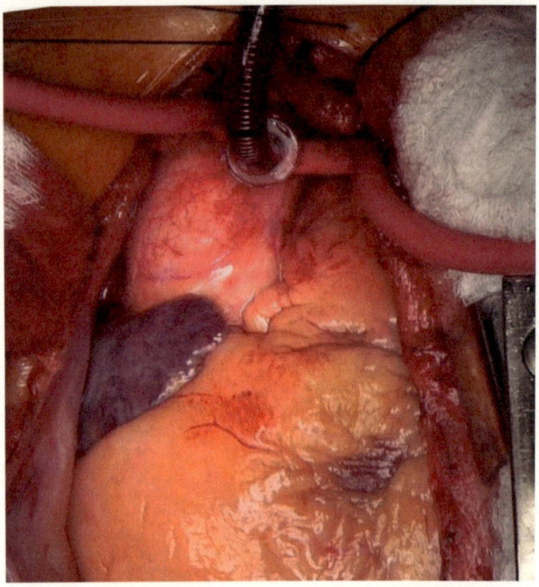

Figure 5.
The aortic cannula has been inserted, and the purse string sutures snared down.

or figure-of-eight suture can be placed to reinforce the aortotomy [12]. The use of felt pledges is left to the discretion of the surgeon. These are composed of prosthetic material such as polytetrafluorethylene and are used to achieve a greater level of hemostasis, especially in patients with fragile tissue such as the elderly [12]. There is, however, a theoretically increased risk of bacterial infection with their use [12]. When closing femoral or axillary cannulation sites, a bovine pericardial patch is frequently used so as not to narrow the arterial diameter significantly.

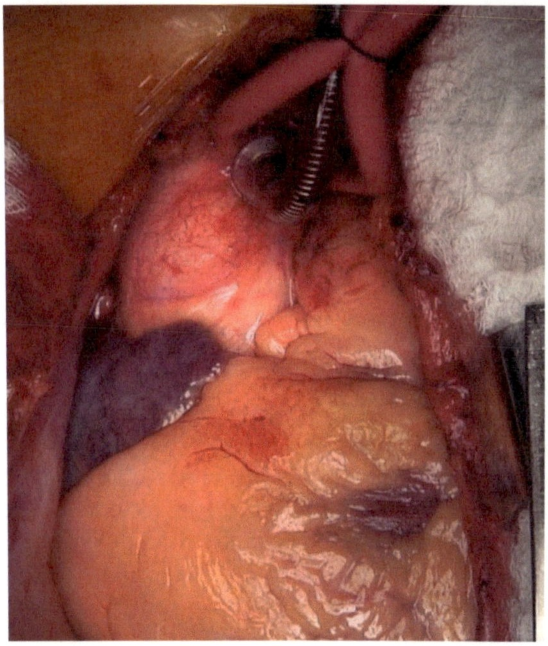

Figure 6.
The aortic cannula and snared purse string sutures are secured together with a heavy silk suture.

7. Axillary artery cannulation

If the axillary artery is selected as the cannulation site, the exposure should be completed prior to median sternotomy. The right side is preferred. To isolate the artery, an incision is made 2 fingerbreadths inferiorly at the middle 1/3 of the clavicle. The incision may be extended laterally. The subcutaneous tissue is dissected down to the level of the pectoralis major. The pectoralis major is then split in the direction of its fibers, and the pecoralis minor is retracted laterally. The axillary vein is the first vascular structure encountered. It is dissected out and retracted inferiorly. Care should be taken to ligate small venous branches. The brachial plexus is superior to the artery and should be avoided if possible. Once the axillary artery is dissected from the surrounding tissue and isolated, the decision must be made to cannulate the artery directly or use an extension graft, such as Dacron. If the artery is to be cannulated directly, open transverse arteriotomy may be made or Seldinger technique employed for cannula placement. A graft is most helpful for small arteries where there is concern that the size of the cannula will completely occlude distal flow or if there is concern that the artery will be significantly narrowed when the arteriotomy is closed. If a graft is to be used, proximal and distal clamps should be placed on the artery, followed by a longitudinal arteriotomy. Graft anastomosis is typically completed with a 6-0 polypropylene suture. After the anastomosis is complete, the graft can be cannulated and blood flow to the arm restored. At the completion of cardiopulmonary bypass, the graft may be ligated and oversewn. If a graft is not used, the arteriotomy can be closed in the standard fashion after decannulation. Standard cannulation strategies should be used, as discussed above. After decannulation, the pectoralis major should be reapproximated so as to cover the arteriotomy, and the incision should be closed in layers [13, 14].

8. Femoral artery cannulation

The femoral artery has long been used for cardiopulmonary bypass since the advent of cardiac surgery. As mentioned above, the femoral artery is a good alternative to direct aortic cannulation in the setting of porcelain aorta, type A aortic dissection, and re-operative cardiac surgery, as well as minimally invasive cardiac procedures [15–17]. The femoral artery can be cannulated percutaneously or directly. An extension graft is almost never needed for femoral cannulation, as opposed to axillary artery cannulation.

Several commercial sets are available to assist in percutaneous cannulation. A percutaneous cannulation is unlikely to be successful in patients who do not have a palpable femoral pulse. To start, the femoral artery should be identified by palpation or ultrasound guidance. The common femoral artery should be punctured well above the superficial/profunda femoral artery bifurcation so as to decrease the incidence of limb malperfusion. Seldinger technique is then employed to completed cannulation. When using femoral artery cannulation for aortic dissection, it is vital to identify the guide wire in the true lumen by TEE prior to cannula placement. Closure preferences for the arteriotomy vary. Several commercial closure devices are available, such as Perclose Proglide Vascular Closure Device (Abbott Inc., Santa Clara, CA) [18]. The field of endovascular closure devices is rapidly growing due to the popularity of endovascular procedures such as abdominal aortic aneurysm repair and transcatheter valve replacement. If the arteriotomy is not hemostatic after attempted endovascular closure and prolonged pressure, a femoral cutdown may be necessary for direct surgical closure of the artery.

For open surgical femoral artery cannulation, an incision should be made parallel to the inguinal crease. The subcutaneous tissues should be dissected down until the femoral artery can be identified and isolated. Proximal and distal control is obtained, and the common femoral artery can be directly cannulated. At the termination of cardiopulmonary bypass, the artery is the repaired directly, typically with 4-0 or 5-0 polypropylene suture. Femoral approach, both percutaneous and via cutdown, can be significantly more difficult to successfully perform on obese patients and patients with severe peripheral vascular disease.

9. Intraoperative techniques and imaging

Patients undergoing cardiopulmonary bypass are at risk for developing neurological deficits due to the dislodgement of atheroma from the aorta and proximal arch during the procedure [19]. Therefore, it is imperative that these atheromas are identified accurately to avoid the development of such complications. The standard method for detecting atherosclerotic disease of the aorta intraoperatively is manual palpation performed by the surgeon [20]. However, it has been noted that this traditional technique is unable to detect approximately 50% of atheroma lesions due to the presence of soft calcifications that the surgeon cannot appropriately identify [21].

An imaging modality that is routinely utilized in cardiac procedures is intraoperative transesophageal echocardiogram (TEE). TEE has shown to be effective in identifying areas of the aorta that are affected by atherosclerotic disease [10].

However, this method is not comprehensive as the bronchus creates a blind spot due to its position between the aorta and esophagus [19].

The best approach to identifying the presence of atheroma lesions in the aorta and proximal arch is epi-aortic scanning. This method involves directly imaging the aortic root and arch via ultrasound. An investigation conducted by Syliviris and colleagues [21] found that epi-aortic scanning was superior to both palpation and TEE in both identifying areas of atherosclerosis and grading the lesions.

Once the locations of atheroma lesions have been identified, modifications to the surgical approach can be made in order to ensure appropriate cannulation and clamping sites. Avoidance of these diseased locations will help to decrease the likelihood of neurologic complications due to disruption of the atherosclerotic regions.

10. Arterial cannulation site complications

10.1 Bleeding

Intraoperative bleeding can be a painful complication for both the surgeon and the patient. Bleeding from the aortic cannulation site is most commonly from too large of an aortotomy or inadequate snaring of the purse string sutures. To prevent this, careful attention should be paid to the diameter of the purse string "circle" that is created to ensure that it is 3–5 mm wider than the cannula diameter, typically 1.5–2 cm in total diameter. It can be challenging to place an additional circumferential suture after the aortotomy has been made. Additionally, care should be taken when making the aortotomy that the scalpel is not inserted too deeply so as to injure the posterior wall of the ascending aorta.

10.2 Malposition of cannula tip

Monitor circuit and peripheral arterial line mean arterial pressures to ensure adequate systemic circulation. Unequal mean arterial pressures suggests cannula malposition, which can typically be corrected by slightly withdrawing the cannula while taking care not to withdraw the cannula completely. Circuit flow rates should be maintained around 2.4 $L/min/m^2$ to ensure cerebral perfusion. If the flow rates are decreased, cannula position should be verified both visually and with intraoperative TEE.

10.3 Embolic events

Visual inspection and palpation of the distal ascending aorta prior to cannulation is of utmost importance in preventing embolic events. A calcified aortic wall is more likely to cause not only difficulty in successfully inserting an aortic cannula but also showering of plaque to the systemic circulation. In addition, intraoperative TEE and epi-aortic ultrasound can be employed to help select an adequate cannulation site for complex aortic walls. If a heavy calcified porcelain aorta is present but not appreciated on preoperative imaging (which would be rare), alternate cannulation sites should be considered. A caveat to this is that atherosclerotic disease that majorly affects the aorta is also likely to affect femoral or axillary vessels.

10.4 Aortic dissection

Aortic dissection is the most feared complication related to aortic cannulation. If not promptly recognized and addressed, the effects can be devastating. Placement of the cannula into the true aortic lumen, as detailed above using adequate pressure gradient monitoring in the bypass circuit, sufficient blood return in the cannula after placement, and verification of placement with TEE significantly decrease the risk of dissection. Atherosclerotic plaques can tear between the medial and intimal layers causing dissection if a cannula is attempted to be forced though a calcified area on the aortic wall. In addition, severe hypertension after decannulation when the aortic purse string sutures are being tied down can lead to tears in the aortic wall layers [3, 22, 23].

11. Conclusion

Cardiac surgery has undergone significant progress over the last 65 years that would not have been possible without the evolution of cardiopulmonary bypass. Several strategies, tips, and pitfalls have been presented above to provide the greatest opportunity for successful arterial cannulation for bypass.

Author details

Emily Bond, Crystal Valadon and Mark Slaughter*
University of Louisville Department of Cardiothoracic Surgery, Louisville, Kentucky, United States

*Address all correspondence to: mark.slaughter@louisville.edu

References

[1] Hessel EA. A brief history of cardiopulmonary bypass. Seminars in Cardiothoracic and Vascular Anesthesia. 2014;**18**(2):87-100. DOI: 10.1177/1089253214530045

[2] Hickey P, Buckley M, Philbin D. Pulsatile and nonpulsatile cardiopulmonary bypass: Review of a counterproductive controversy. The Annals of Thoracic Surgery. 1983;**36**(6):720-737

[3] Kincaid EH, Hammon JW. Cardiopulmonary bypass. In: Yuh DD, Vricella LA, Yang SC, Doty JR, editors. Johns Hopkins Textbook of Cardiothoracic Surgery. 2nd ed. New York, NY: McGraw-Hill; 2014

[4] El-Sherief AH, Wu CC, Schoenhagen P, Little BP, Cheng A, Abbara S, et al. Basics of cardiopulmonary bypass: Normal and abnormal postoperative CT appearances. Radiographics. 2013;**33**:63-72. DOI: 10.1148/rg.331115747

[5] Ramchandani M, Al Jabbari O, Abu Saleh WK, Ramlawi B. Cannulation strategies and pitfalls in minimally invasive cardiac surgery. Methodist DeBakey Cardiovascular Journal. 2016;**12**(1):10-13

[6] Cantinotti, M. The importance and ways of exploring the entire chest before and after cardiac surgery: Chest radiography, lung ultrasonography, and computed tomography. The Journal of Thoracic and Cardiovascular Surgery. 2018;**155**(5):2041-2042

[7] LaPar DJ, Ailawadi G, et al. Preoperative computed tomography is associated with lower risk of perioperative stroke in reoperative cardiac surgery. Interactive CardioVascular and Thoracic Surgery. 2011;**12**(6):919-923. DOI: 10.1510/icvts.2010.265165

[8] Qizilbash B, Couture P, Denault A. Impact of perioperative transesophageal echocardiography in aortic valve replacement. Seminars in Cardiothoracic and Vascular Anesthesia. 2017;**11**(4):288-300. DOI: 10.1177/1089253207311789

[9] Patel A, Kannam J. Transesophageal Echocardiography: Indications, Complications, and Normal Views. UpToDate. Retrieved from: https://www.uptodate.com/contents/transesophageal-echocardiography-indications-complications-and-normal-views

[10] Hessel EA, Hill AG. Circuitry and cannulation techniques. In: Gravlee GP, Davis RF, Kursz M, Utley JR, editors. Cardiopulmonary Bypass: Principles and Practice. 2nd ed. Philadelphia, PA: LWW; 2000

[11] Kwon MH, Tollis G, Sundt TM. Myocardial revascularization with cardiopulmonary bypass. In: Cohn LH, Adams DH, editors. Cardiac Surgery in the Adult. 5th ed. New York, NY: McGraw-Hill; 2018

[12] Tappainer E. A stitch in time saves nine: Closing the hole after removal of the aortic root cannula. Journal of Cardiothoracic Surgery. 2009;**4**:2. DOI: 10.1186/1749-8090-4-2

[13] Valentine RJ. Surgical treatment of the subclavian and axillary artery. In: Chaifkof EL, Cambria RP, editors. Atlas of Vascular Surgery and Endovascular Therapy. 1st ed. Philadelphia: Saunders; 2014. pp. 157-170

[14] Sinclair MC, Singer RL, Manley NJ, Montesano CCP. Cannulation of the axillary artery for cardiopulmonary bypass: Safeguards and pitfalls. The Annals of Thoracic Surgery. 2003;**75**:931-934. DOI: 10.1016/S0003-4975(02)04497-1

[15] Ayyash B, Tranquilli M, Elefteriades JA. Femoral artery cannulation for thoracic aortic surgery: Safe under transesophageal echocardiographic control. The Journal of Thoracic and Cardiovascular Surgery. 2011;**142**:1478-1481

[16] Schwarz B, Mair P, Margreiter J, et al. Experience with percutaneous venoarterial cardiopulmonary bypass for emergency circulatory support. Critical Care Medicine. 2003;**31**:758-764

[17] Fusco DS, Shaw RK, Tranquilli M, Kopf GS, Eleteriades JA. Femoral cannulation is safe for type A dissection repair. The Annals of Thoracic Surgery. 2004;**78**:1285-1289

[18] Yang L, Liu J, Li Y. Femoral artery closure versus surgical cutdown for endovascular aortic repair: A single-center experience. Medical Science Monitor. 2018;**24**:92-99. DOI: 10.12659/MSM.905350

[19] Joo H-C, Youn Y-N, Kwak Y-L, Yi G-J, Yoo K-J. Intraoperative epiaortic scanning for preventing early stroke after off-pump coronary artery bypass. BJA: British Journal of Anaesthesia. 2013;**111**(3):374-381. DOI: 10.1093/bja/aet113

[20] Katz E, Tunick P, Facc H, et al. Protruding aortic atheromas predict stroke in elderly patients undergoing cardiopulmonary bypass: Experience with intraoperative transesophageal echocardiography. Journal of the American College of Cardiology. 1992;**20**(1):70-77

[21] Sylivris S, Calafiore P, Matalanis G, et al. The intraoperative assessment of ascending aortic atheroma: Epiaortic imaging is superior to both transesophageal echocardiography and direct palpation. Journal of Cardiothoracic and Vascular Anesthesia. 1997;**11**:704-707. DOI: 10.1016/S1053-0770(97)90161-0

[22] Williams C, Suwansirikul S, Engelman R. Thoracic aortic dissection following cannulation for perfusion. The Annals of Thoracic Surgery. 1974;**18**(3):300-304

[23] Still R, Hilgenber A, Akins C, et al. Intraoperative aortic dissection. Annals of Thoracic Surgery. 1992;**53**:374-380

Chapter 3

Tips and Pitfalls in Robotic Mitral Valve Surgery

Takashi Murashita

Abstract

Robotic mitral valve repair is now routinely and safely performed all over the world. There are many literatures which showed advantages of reduced blood loss, lower risk of infection, lower risk of atrial fibrillation, shorter length of hospital stay, quicker return to normal activities, and a superior cosmetic result, compared with a conventional sternotomy. However, the introduction of new technique requires a learning curve even for expert mitral valve surgeons. There are complications specifically related to robotic mitral valve surgery, such as major vascular complications, inadequate myocardial protection, and unilateral pulmonary edema. The purpose of this chapter is to characterize the tips and pitfalls of robotic mitral valve repair and to discuss the controversial issues in the contemporary practice.

Keywords: robotic surgery, mitral valve repair, complication

1. Introduction

Since the introduction of robotic mitral valve repair in the late 1990s, the number of this procedure has been increasing worldwide. Many centers have reported excellent outcomes of robotic mitral valve repair [1–8]. In the beginning, it was mainly applied in selected patients with a simple repair case and relatively low risk cases. However, with the accumulation of surgical experience, the indication has been broadened to complicated repair cases or aged patients.

Wang et al. reviewed the Society of Thoracic Surgeons database and compared surgical outcomes of robotic and surgical mitral valve repair in patients aged 65 years and older [9]. They found that robotic mitral valve repair was associated with less postoperative atrial fibrillation, less blood transfusion, and shorter intensive care unit and hospital stay compared with surgical mitral valve repair without a difference in 3-year mortality, heart failure readmission, or mitral valve reintervention.

2. Tips and pitfalls

2.1 Applying to a robot platform

Robotic mitral valve repair is usually done thorough a right thoracotomy; thus, intra-thoracic pathology such as previous right thoracotomy, severe pulmonary dysfunction, and chest deformity can be a contraindication [10]. Patients at risk for coronary artery disease should undergo a cardiac catheterization, and severe coronary artery disease requiring coronary artery bypass grafting is another contraindication of robotic mitral valve repair. In addition, significant pulmonary hypertension or severe right ventricular dysfunction is included to contraindications.

Usually, robotic mitral valve repair is done with a 5- to 6-cm right thoracotomy [11]. A specific attention should be paid for inserting robotic instruments into the right chest. The insertion of service ports can injure the right lung, vessels, diaphragm, liver, and mediastinal structures. **Figure 1** shows our regular setup for robotic instruments. The thoracotomy is made through fourth or fifth intercostal space. We carefully review the preoperative computer tomography and decide which intercostal space would give us the best exposure for mitral valve. The port for left arm is usually inserted through second or third intercostal space. The port for left atrial retractor is usually inserted through the same intercostal space with thoracotomy. The port for right arm is usually inserted through sixth or seventh intercostal space. The camera port is inserted one higher intercostal space than thoracotomy.

2.2 The interaction between the operator and the assistance

After the robotic instruments are inserted, the surgeon moves to the robotic console, and the assistant will move to the patient's right side and has an access to the operative field through the thoracotomy. From the console, the surgeons can perform precise movements inside the heart using the mechanical instruments. The mechanical instruments include forceps, scissors, needle holders, and electrocautery. The surgeons use two mechanical instruments, and the changes of the instruments were manipulated by the bedside assistant.

The role of the surgeon on console is to accomplish a mitral valve repair by cutting, suturing, and sizing with two mechanical instruments, whereas, the role of bedside assistant is suctioning the field, suture following, and knot tying. Since the operative field is very limited, the bedside assistant should be trained for knot-tying instruments.

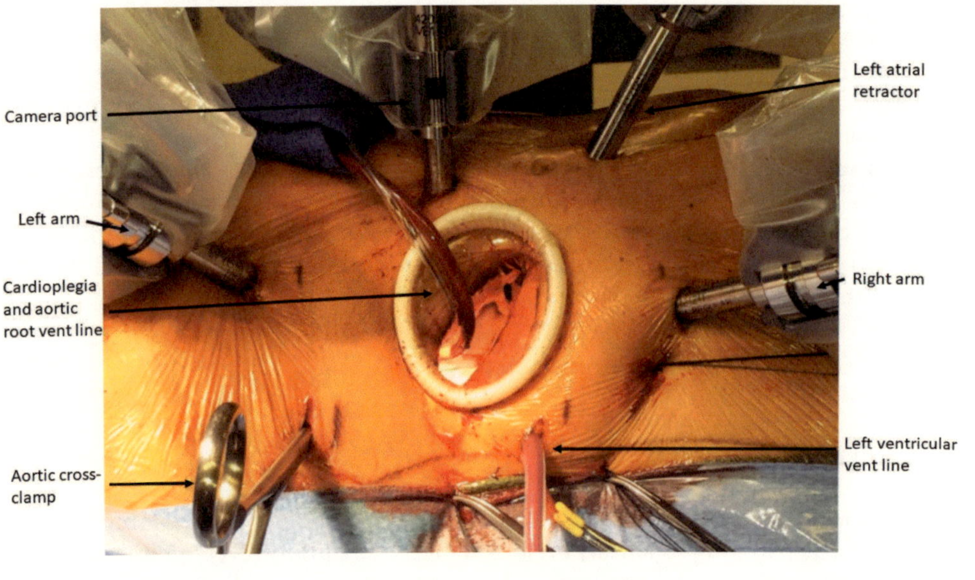

Figure 1.
The picture of a standard setup for robotic mitral valve surgery.

DOI: http://dx.doi.org/10.5772/intechopen.85241

2.3 Establishment of a cardiopulmonary bypass

In a robotic mitral valve repair, cardiopulmonary bypass is established either via an antegrade perfusion with a central cannulation or via a retrograde perfusion with a peripheral cannulation. It is a controversy in which perfusion strategy is optimal [12].

Murzi et al. reviewed 1421 patients who underwent antegrade perfusion and 141 patients who underwent retrograde perfusion [13]. They reported that retrograde perfusion was associated with higher incidence of stroke than antegrade perfusion (3.5 vs. 1.1%). In the meantime, LaPietra et al. reviewed 1501 patients, and found that stroke rate was low (about 1.5%) regardless of cannulation technique [14]. Nowadays, several experienced centers routinely apply retrograde femoral perfusion during minimally invasive mitral valve surgery [1, 3, 6].

In establishing the peripheral cannulation, the venous drainage for cardiopulmonary bypass is obtained by a placement of cannula, usually via the right femoral vein and right internal jugular vein. It is essential to introduce cannula under a transesophageal echocardiography to avoid the risk of extravasation, migration of the cannula, or other types of complications [15]. Arterial cannula is usually inserted to the right femoral artery. It is also essential to obtain a preoperative multidetector computed tomography angiography for the assessment of aortoiliac atherosclerosis in order to plan an optimal surgical approach [16].

2.4 Aortic cross-clamp

For aortic cross-clamp, there are basically two options: endoaortic or transthoracic clamp (**Figure 2**). The endoaortic cross-clamp is performed with an

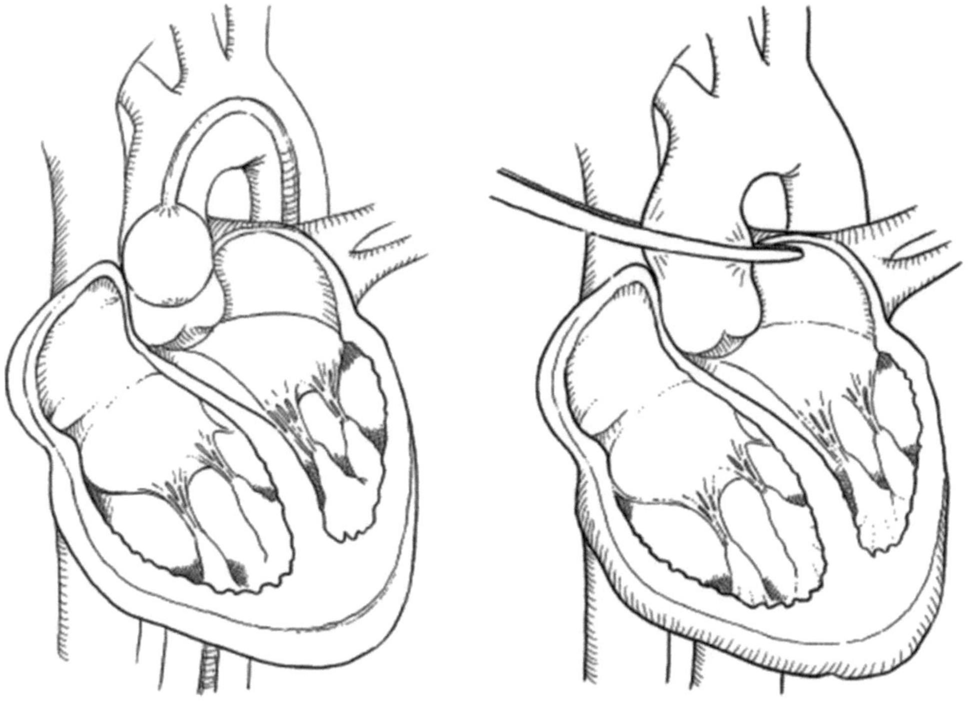

Figure 2.
Left: endoaortic cross-clamping with an endoaortic balloon. Right: transthoracic cross-clamping using a Chitwood clamp.

endoaortic balloon, which comprises a triple lumen catheter mostly introduced usually through a left femoral artery with an inflatable balloon at the tip. The central lumen is used for delivery of cardioplegia and aortic root vent. The remaining lumen is used for balloon inflation and deflation as well as pressure monitoring. The transthoracic clamp is called Chitwood clamp, and is introduced through the intercostal space and positioned around the aorta.

Maselli et al. monitored embolic events with a transcranial Doppler during minimally invasive mitral valve surgery, and found that brain embolism occurred predominantly at the time of ascending aorta clamping and declamping with an endoaortic balloon [17]. In the meantime, the application of an external cross-clamp to the ascending aorta may cause the embolic events and traumatic injury.

The superiority between two methods of aortic cross-clamp has been controversial.

Kowalewski et al. performed a meta-analysis of observational studies [18]. They found that there was no difference of cerebrovascular events, all-cause mortality, and kidney injury between endoaortic and transthoracic cross-clamp; however, endoaortic balloon occlusion was associated with a higher risk of iatrogenic aortic dissection (0.93 vs. 0.13%) and higher risk of leg ischemia (0.47 vs. 0.20%) than transthoracic cross-clamp.

Kesavuori et al. reported their initial 5-year results of robotic mitral valve repairs [19]. The postoperative complications included conversion to sternotomy, reoperations for bleeding, and low cardiac output states requiring extracorporeal membrane oxygenation. They reported that early major robotic complications were related to the use of endoaortic balloon occlusion.

In the meantime, Barbero et al. reviewed three centers' experience of minimally invasive mitral valve surgery, and did not find differences in respiratory failure, major vascular complication, stroke, and in-hospital mortality between endoaortic and transthoracic aortic clamping [20].

2.5 Myocardial protection

Although several ways of myocardial protection have been advocated in minimally invasive mitral valve surgery, the optimal method has been controversial. There is a choice of antegrade or retrograde, intermittent or continuous, and crystalloid or blood cardioplegia.

One of the earliest approaches were antegrade cardioplegia via the endoaortic balloon, as described in the "aortic cross-clamp." Lebon et al. compared 118 patients undergoing minimally invasive mitral valve surgery and 118 patients undergoing open mitral valve surgery, and found no difference in the incidence of difficult weaning from bypass and intra-aortic balloon pump use between two groups [21].

When applying transthoracic cross-clamp, direct cardioplegia insertion into the ascending aorta through a long antegrade cardioplegia catheter is necessary. As the insertion site of cardioplegia catheter gets far in the thoracotomy, the insertion and decannulation of the catheter can be associated with higher risk of bleeding than sternotomy.

In the setting of aortic insufficiency, retrograde cardioplegia might be desirable. Retrograde cardioplegia can be performed by placement of a percutaneous coronary sinus catheter via the internal jugular vein, but that requires specialized skills with an increased cost of a specialized catheter. In addition, the retrograde cardioplegia catheter insertion can cause catheter displacement, coronary sinus rupture, and inadequate protection of the right ventricle [22]. Another option of retrograde cardioplegia is to directly insert a catheter through a purse-string in the right atrium under a transesophageal echocardiography.

There are two types of cardioplegia solution: crystalloid and blood. Blood cardioplegia is usually chosen in the open-heart surgery, as it has two advantages over pure crystalloid cardioplegia. First, blood cardioplegia can deliver oxygen to the myocardium, and secondly, the additional crystalloid volume is small; thus, hemodilution or myocardial edema can be avoided. Therefore, some centers still use blood cardioplegia in minimally invasive mitral valve surgery.

However, some centers prefer crystalloid-based cardioplegia: histidine-tryptophan-ketoglutarate cardioplegia [19, 23]. The advantage of this cardioplegia is that a single antegrade shot can maintain adequate myocardial protection up to 2 hours; thus, potentially aortic cross-clamp time and cardiopulmonary bypass time can be reduced.

2.6 Unilateral pulmonary edema

Unilateral pulmonary edema is known as an uncommon, but frequently lethal complication following minimally invasive robotic cardiac surgery. The clinical presentation of this condition includes severe right lung edema developing within the first several minutes to hours after coming off from a cardiopulmonary bypass (**Figure 3**), which leads to profound hypoxia, hypercapnia, pulmonary hypertension, and hemodynamic instability.

The mechanism of this condition is yet to be fully understood. Lung deflation is shown to be associated with the sequestration of inflammatory response. Minamiya et al. reported that during atelectasis, polymorphonuclear leukocytes accumulate in

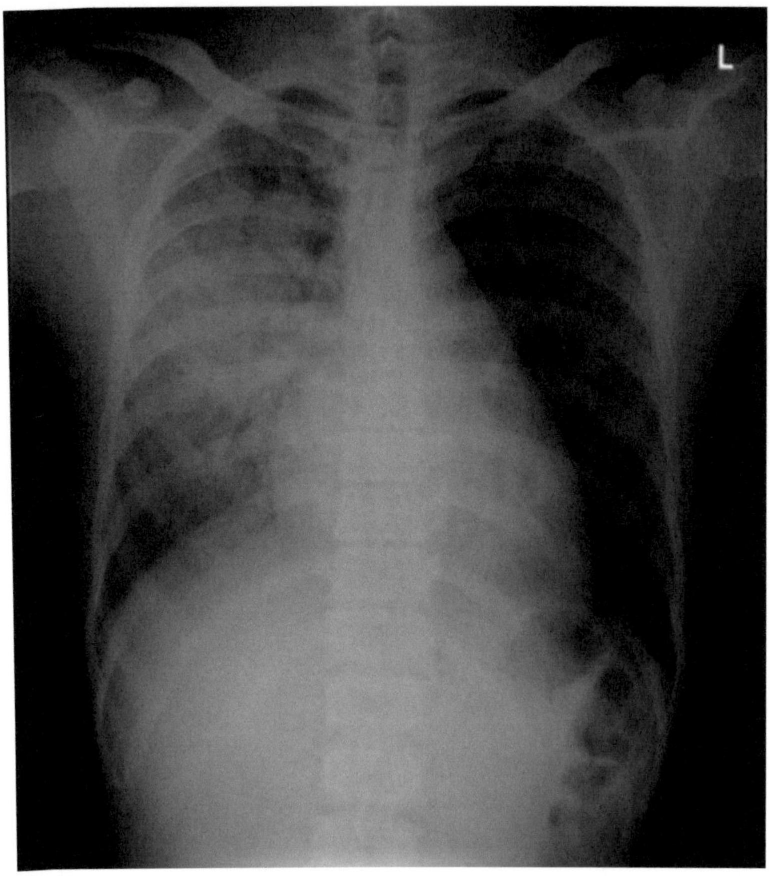

Figure 3.
A typical chest X-ray imaging showing unilateral pulmonary edema on the right side.

the lung, and after pulmonary reexpansion, polymorphonuclear leukocytes respiratory bursting occurs [24]. The inflammatory response may be aggravated by the use of cardiopulmonary bypass. It is reported that prolonged cardiopulmonary bypass time and lung collapse are associated with the occurrence of unilateral pulmonary edema. Other factors such as obesity and intraoperative blood product use may affect the inflammatory response.

Renner et al. reviewed their 256 patients who underwent minimally invasive mitral valve surgery, and they encountered five cases (2.0%) of unilateral pulmonary edema, which required postoperative extracorporeal membrane oxygenation; two of them had in-hospital mortality [25]. They reported that preoperative high C-reactive protein and long cardiopulmonary bypass time were associated with the occurrence of unilateral pulmonary edema.

Irisawa et al. reviewed 381 patients who underwent minimally invasive cardiac surgery, and found 8 (2.1%) patients developed unilateral pulmonary edema [26]. They reported that preoperative use of steroid or immunosuppressive drugs and prolonged aortic cross-clamp time were the risk factors for unilateral pulmonary edema.

Keyl et al. reported that the use of dexamethasone significantly reduced the incidence of unilateral pulmonary edema from 12.9 to 4.0% [27]. Moss et al. reported their modifications to the robotic mitral valve repair technique in an effort to reduce the incidence of unilateral pulmonary edema [28]. They hypothesized that unilateral pulmonary edema results from severe right lung ischemia due to insufficient bronchial artery flow. Their modifications were focused on right lung oxygen supply, and included minimization of right rung deflation before cardiopulmonary bypass, infusion of unheated CO2 into the right chest, active cooling to low systemic temperature, maintaining high mean arterial pressure during cardiopulmonary bypass, and restoration of right lung ventilation was early as possible.

3. Conclusions

Although many reports demonstrated the efficacy and safety of robotic mitral valve repair, there are some specific pitfalls, which surgeons do not encounter in a conventional open heart surgery. In order to achieve a good success of robotic mitral valve repair, surgeons need to understand these particular issues and avoid robotic-related complications.

Author details

Takashi Murashita
University of Missouri, One Hospital Drive, Columbia, Missouri, USA

*Address all correspondence to: tmurashita@gmail.com

References

[1] Gillinov AM, Mihaljevic T, Javadikasgari H, Suri RM, Mick SL, Navia JL, et al. Early results of robotically assisted mitral valve surgery: Analysis of the first 1000 cases. The Journal of Thoracic and Cardiovascular Surgery. 2018;**155**:82-91. DOI: 10.1016/j.jtcvs.2017.07.037

[2] Javadikasgari H, Suri RM, Tappuni B, Lowry AM, Mihaljevic T, Mick S, et al. Robotic mitral valve repair for degenerative posterior leaflet prolapse. Annals of Cardiothoracic Surgery. 2017;**6**:27-32. DOI: 10.21037/acs.2017.01.07

[3] Kim HJ, Kim JB, Jung SH, Lee JW. Clinical outcomes of robotic mitral valve repair: A single-center experience in Korea. Annals of Cardiothoracic Surgery, 2017;**6**:9-16. DOI: 10.21037/acs.2016.10.02

[4] Mihaljevic T, Jarrett CM, Gillinov AM, Williams SJ, DeVilliers PA, Stewart WJ, et al. Robotic repair of posterior mitral valve prolapse versus conventional approaches: Potential realized. The Journal of Thoracic and Cardiovascular Surgery. 2011;**141**:72-80. DOI: 10.1016/j.jtcvs.2010.09.008

[5] Navarra E, Mastrobuoni S, De Kerchove L, Glineur D, Watremez C, Van Dyck M, et al. Robotic mitral valve repair: A European single-centre experience. Interactive Cardiovascular and Thoracic Surgery. 2017;**25**:62-67. DOI: 10.1093/icvts/ivx060

[6] Ramzy D, Trento A, Cheng W, De Robertis MA, Mirocha J, Ruzza A, et al. Three hundred robotic-assisted mitral valve repairs: The cedars-Sinai experience. The Journal of Thoracic and Cardiovascular Surgery. 2014;**147**:228-235. DOI: 10.1016/j.jtcvs.2013.09.035

[7] Suri RM, Taggarse A, Burkhart HM, Daly RC, Mauermann W, Nishimura RA, et al. Robotic mitral valve repair for simple and complex degenerative disease: Midterm clinical and echocardiographic quality outcomes. Circulation. 2015;**132**:1961-1968. DOI: 10.1161/CIRCULATIONAHA.115.017792

[8] Murphy DA, Moss E, Binongo J, Miller JS, Macheers SK, Sarin EL, et al. The expanding role of endoscopic robotics in mitral valve surgery: 1,257 consecutive procedures. The Annals of Thoracic Surgery. 2015;**100**:1675-1681. DOI: 10.1016/j.athoracsur.2015.05.068

[9] Wang A, Brennan JM, Zhang S, Jung SH, Yerokun B, Cox ML, et al. Robotic mitral valve repair in older individuals: An analysis of the Society of Thoracic Surgeons database. The Annals of Thoracic Surgery. 2018;**106**:1388-1393. DOI: 10.1016/j.athoracsur.2018.05.074

[10] Suri RM, Dearani JA, Mihaljevic T, Chitwood WR Jr, Murphy DA, Trento A, et al. Mitral valve repair using robotic technology: Safe, effective, and durable. The Journal of Thoracic and Cardiovascular Surgery. 2016;**151**:1450-1454. DOI: 10.1016/j.jtcvs.2016.02.030

[11] Nifong LW, Chitwood WR, Pappas PS, Smith CR, Argenziano M, Starnes VA, et al. Robotic mitral valve surgery: A United States multicenter trial. The Journal of Thoracic and Cardiovascular Surgery. 2005;**129**:1395-1404

[12] Badhwar V. Are we going backwards or forwards in minimally invasive mitral valve surgery? Three eras of perfusion strategy. Seminars in Thoracic and Cardiovascular Surgery. 2015;**27**:104-105. DOI: 10.1053/j.semtcvs.2015.09.002

[13] Murzi M, Cerillo AG, Gasbarri T, Margaryan R, Kallushi E, Farneti P, et al. Antegrade and retrograde

perfusion in minimally invasive mitral valve surgery with transthoracic aortic clamping: A single-institution experience with 1632 patients over 12 years. Interactive Cardiovascular and Thoracic Surgery. 2017;**24**:363-368. DOI: 10.1093/icvts/ivw370

[14] LaPietra A, Santana O, Mihos CG, DeBeer S, Rosen GP, Lamas GA, et al. Incidence of cerebrovascular accidents in patients undergoing minimally invasive valve surgery. The Journal of Thoracic and Cardiovascular Surgery. 2014;**148**:156-160. DOI: 10.1016/j.jtcvs.2013.08.016

[15] Rehfeldt KH, Andre JV, Ritter MJ. Anesthetic considerations in robotic mitral valve surgery. Annals of Cardiothoracic Surgery. 2017;**6**:47-53. DOI: 10.21037/acs.2017.01.10

[16] Moodley S, Schoenhagen P, Gillinov AM, Mihaljevic T, Flamm SD, Griffin BP, et al. Preoperative multidetector computed tomograpy angiography for planning of minimally invasive robotic mitral valve surgery: Impact on decision making. The Journal of Thoracic and Cardiovascular Surgery. 2013;**146**:262-268. DOI: 10.1016/j.jtcvs.2012.06.052

[17] Maselli D, Pizio R, Musumeci F. Multifrequency transcranial Doppler for intraoperative automatic detection and characterisation of cerebral microemboli during port-access mitral valve surgery. Interactive Cardiovascular and Thoracic Surgery. 2006;**5**:32-35

[18] Kowalewski M, Malvindi PG, Suwalski P, Raffa GM, Pawliszak W, Perlinski D, et al. Clinical safety and effectiveness of endoaortic as compared to transthoracic clamp for small thoracotomy mitral valve surgery: Meta-analysis of observational studies. The Annals of Thoracic Surgery. 2017;**103**:676-686. DOI: 10.1016/j.athoracsur.2016.08.072

[19] Kesävuori R, Raivio P, Jokinen JJ, Sahlman A, Teittinen K, Vento A. Early experience with robotic mitral valve repair with intra-aortic occlusion. The Journal of Thoracic and Cardiovascular Surgery. 2018;**155**:1463-1471. DOI: 10.1016/j.jtcvs.2017.10.076

[20] Barbero C, Krakor R, Bentala M, Casselman F, Candolfi P, Goldstein J, et al. Comparison of endoaortic and transthoracic aortic clamping in less-invasive mitral valve surgery. The Annals of Thoracic Surgery. 2018;**105**:794-798. DOI: 10.1016/j.athoracsur.2017.09.054

[21] Lebon JS, Couture P, Fortier A, Rochon AG, Ayoub C, Viens C, et al. Myocardial protection in mitral valve surgery: Comparison between minimally invasive approach and standard Sternotomy. Journal of Cardiothoracic and Vascular Anesthesia. 2018;**32**:656-663. DOI: 10.1053/j.jvca.2017.08.040

[22] Bainbridge D, Fernandes P, Chu MWA. Cardioplegia during minimally invasive mitral valve surgery, a team approach. Journal of Cardiothoracic and Vascular Anesthesia. 2018;**32**:664-665. DOI: 10.1053/j.jvca.2017.10.012

[23] Garbade J, Davierwala P, Seeburger J, Pfannmueller B, Misfeld M, Borger MA, et al. Myocardial protection during minimally invasive mitral valve surgery: Strategies and cardioplegic solutions. Annals of Cardiothoracic Surgery. 2013;**2**:803-808. DOI: 10.3978/j.issn.2225-319X.2013.09.04

[24] Minamiya Y, Saito H, Takahashi N, Kawai H, Ito M, Hosono Y, et al. Polymorphonuclear leukocytes are activated during atelectasis before lung reexpansion in rat. Shock. 2008;**30**:81-86. DOI: 10.1097/SHK.0b013e31815dd221

[25] Renner J, Lorenzen U, Borzikowsky C, Schoeneich F, Cremer J,

Haneya A, et al. Unilateral pulmonary oedema after minimally invasive mitral valve surgery: A single-centre experience. European Journal of Cardio-Thoracic Surgery. 2018;**53**:764-770. DOI: 10.1093/ejcts/ezx399

[26] Irisawa Y, Hiraoka A, Totsugawa T, Chikazawa G, Nakajima K, Tamura K, et al. Re-expansion pulmonary oedema after minimally invasive cardiac surgery with right mini-thoracotomy. European Journal of Cardio-Thoracic Surgery. 2016;**49**:500-505. DOI: 10.1093/ejcts/ezv089

[27] Keyl C, Staier K, Pingpoh C, Pache G, Thoma M, Günkel L, et al. Unilateral pulmonary oedema after minimally invasive cardiac surgery via right anterolateral minithoracotomy. European Journal of Cardio-Thoracic Surgery. 2015;**47**:1097-1102. DOI: 10.1093/ejcts/ezu312

[28] Moss E, Halkos ME, Binongo JN, Murphy DA. Prevention of unilateral pulmonary edema complicating robotic mitral valve operations. The Annals of Thoracic Surgery. 2017;**103**:98-104. DOI: 10.1016/j.athoracsur.2016.05.100

Chapter 4

Aortic Root Reconstruction

Salah E. Altarabsheh, Salil V. Deo and Yakov E. Elgudin

Abstract

Aortic root reconstruction represents one of the most complex areas of cardiac surgery as well as one of the most dynamic-major developments in understanding of the aortic root anatomy and physiology, improvements in imaging and surgical technique allowed for development and acceptance into clinical practice of several novel procedures over last couple of decades. From first aortic root replacement reported by Bentall and De Bono in 1968 to aortic root reimplantation (David procedure) and remodeling (Yacoub operation) with multiple contemporary modifications, aortic root reconstruction now is widely used in treatment of chronic aortic aneurysmal disease and acute aortic dissections alike. Basic principles of aortic root structure and function and critical operative strategies for aortic root surgery are reviewed in this chapter.

Keywords: aortic root, aneurysm, replacement, reimplantation, remodeling, dissection

1. Introduction

The technique of aortic root surgery has undergone many improvements during the past decades. These are a direct result of better understanding of the functional hemodynamics of the aortic root coupled with significant improvement in imaging. We present here a brief overview of pathology involving the aortic root with a special focus on the surgical aspects in these operative procedures. Our chapter includes tips on use of mechanical valve conduits, homograft, and stent-less valve prostheses as well as techniques implementing a valve-sparing approach.

2. Anatomy and physiology of the aortic root

Improved imaging and computer simulation has increased our understanding of the aortic root anatomy, structure and function. Aortic root had been described as the vascular tube supporting the aortic valve leaflets and connecting the left ventricular outflow tract inferiorly to the sinotubular junction superiorly [1]. Two thirds of the lower segment (aortic annulus) of the aortic root is attached to the interventricular septum while the remainder is attached to the fibrous part of the anterior mitral valve leaflet [2]. This tubular structure (**Figure 1**) encompasses the aortic valve leaflets, coronary ostia, commissures, interleaflet triangles and the sinuses [1]. All these components link together to act as a single unit. It is now clear, that this is much more than just a passive unit governed by pressure changes across the valve [3, 4]. The geometric relationship of the valve leaflets as well as individual lengths are important for it to work as a single efficient hemodynamic unit [5].

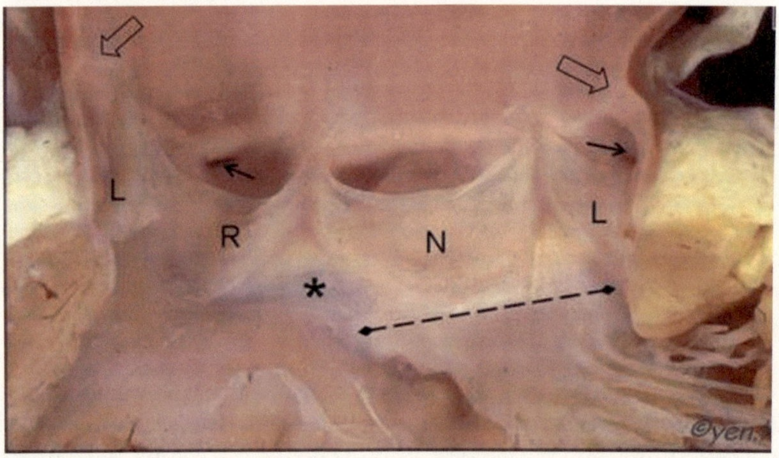

Figure 1.
Opened aortic root section. Sinotubular junction is indicated by the open arrows, small arrows indicating the coronary ostia (left and right), broken lines indicating the fibrous skeleton between the aortic and mitral valves. L, R, and N mark the left, right and the non-coronary cusps, respectively [6].

The dilated portion of the aortic wall between the aortic annulus and sino-tubular junction is known as the sinus of Valsalva. These sinuses are named according to the relationship of the origin of the coronary ostia from the root that is left, right or non-coronary sinuses. The sinuses are labelled corresponding to their coronary ostia. One of the important roles provided by these sinuses is preventing obstruction of the coronary ostia during movement of the aortic valve leaflets against the aortic wall, so that coronary blood flow is maintained [5]. An important function is prevention of ostial obstruction during systole when the aortic valve is open [7]. Generation of Eddy currents during early systole prevents the aortic leaflets from touching the aortic wall [8].

The aortic valve leaflets which are inserted at their bases in a semilunar fashion to the aortic annulus. They allow uni-directional flow of blood from the left ventricle to the aorta. Aortic valve leaflets are variable in size and number, the non-coronary cusp being the largest compared to the left or right aortic valve cusps. The most common variation is the bicuspid aortic valve, which consists of a semi-lunar opening due to the presence of two leaflets, and the commonest deviation from the normal tri-leaflet pattern is the known congenital anomaly called bicuspid aortic valve [9]. The attachment of the curved aortic valve leaflets form the triangular space named as the interleaflet triangles, the apices of these triangles is known as the valve commissures which are at the level of the sinotubular junction [10]. Aortic valve competence depends on the overlap between these adjacent free margins of the leaflets.

The aortic valve annulus represents the ventriculo-aortic junction which is a complex structure and universally accepted term as aortic annulus [9]. The basic attachments of the aortic valve leaflets at the aortic annulus comprise muscular and fibrous parts [5]. The right aortic valve leaflet attaches to both the membranous and the interventricular septa, while the non-coronary leaflet attaches to the membranous septum and the fibrous skeleton of the anterior mitral valve leaflet, and the left aortic valve leaflet attaches to the fibrous skeleton of the anterior mitral valve leaflet and partly to the interventricular septum [9]. Connective tissue disorders that involve the fibrous skeleton of the aortic root lead to alteration in normal geometry. Damage begets further damage leading to significant valve distortion and subsequent clinical sequelae [9].

3. Aortic root pathology

3.1 Connective tissue disorders

Connective tissue disorder is among the most common non-infective etiology of aortic root pathology. Marfan's syndrome, Ehlers-Danlos syndrome and Loeys-Dietz syndrome predominantly involve the elastic aortic root [11–13]. Marfan's syndrome is an autosomal dominant disorder characterized by mutation in the gene encoding for fibrillin-1. It leads to cystic medial necrosis and involves all connective tissue containing high percentages of elastin. Disease is multi-systemic; however aortic dissection remains an important cause of mortality [14]. The probability of aortic emergencies increases significantly when transverse aortic diameters is more than 45 mm [15].

Patients with vascular type of the Ehlers-Danlos syndrome are prone to aortic dissection rather than aneurysm, while patients with Loeys-Dietz syndrome are liable to have aortic aneurysm and dissection at younger age [11, 16, 17].

3.2 Bicuspid aortic valve

Bicuspid aortic valve (BAV) is present in 1–2% of the population; almost 40% also have thoracic aortic dilatation at the time of presentation [18].

While the inheritance of BAV is not clearly defined, gene sequence defects leading to aortopathy is more prevalent in this population [19]. Degenerative changes in the tunica media with reduced elastin increases risk of dissection these patients [20, 21].

3.3 Inflammatory etiology

Giant cell arteritis and Takayasu arteritis are rarer causes of aneurysmal dilatation/aortic dissection [22, 23]. While temporal artery involvement is the hallmark of giant cell arteritis, at least 0.15% also had aortic dissection in an autopsy series [22]. Takayasu arteritis on the other hand is an inflammatory disorder that leads to large vessel inflammation characterized by fibrosis and narrowing, which may lead to aneurysmal formation and possible rupture [23]. Corticosteroids are used for acute therapy and surgery is performed once active inflammation subsides [24, 25].

3.4 Cystic medial necrosis

Cystic medial necrosis (CMN) is a pathological term that is characterized by the formation of cyst like lesions in the medial layer of the large arteries with accumulation of basophilic substances [26].

4. Aortic root aneurysm

The American Association of Thoracic Surgeons present following guidelines regarding surgery for the ascending aorta [27]:

a. Surgical repair should be performed when aortic diameter (root or ascending aorta) is 55 mm or more.

b. Surgical repair should be performed when aortic diameter (root or ascending aorta) is 50 mm or more in the presence of certain risk factors such as: root phenotype bicuspid aortic valve, uncontrolled hypertension, history of aortic dissection or sudden death in the family, annual enlargement of 3 mm or more in the size of the aortic aneurysm, or predominantly aortic regurgitation.

c. Surgical repair should be performed when aortic diameter (root or ascending aorta) is 50 mm or more in patients with low operative risk being performed by experienced aortic surgical team in centers with well-established surgical outcomes

d. Surgical repair should be performed when aortic diameter (root or ascending aorta) is 45 mm or more in patients undergoing concomitant other cardiac surgery.

Patients with Marfan's syndrome or Marfanoid habitus should be operated when their aortic root/ascending aorta is larger than 50 mm in maximal transverse diameter [28]. Gott and colleagues [27, 28] reported an improved 30-day survival in a series of 675 patients with Marfan's syndrome who underwent elective compared to urgent or emergency replacement of the aortic root.

If patients have a family history of aortic dissection, demonstrate an annual increase of 3 mm or have significant aortic regurgitation, then aortic root surgery is warranted when diameters exceed 45 mm [29]. Hormonal changes during pregnancy significantly increase risk of aortic dissection. Hence, women of child-bearing age who are keen to have a family are recommended surgery prior to pregnancy. These guidelines are also applicable to patients with Ehlers-Danlos syndrome and Loeys-Dietz syndrome.

5. Sinus of Valsalva aneurysm

Sinus of Valsalva aneurysms are rare; reported in 0.09% of autopsy series [30]. This condition affects commonly the right coronary sinus to a lesser degree the non-coronary sinus; involvement of all three sinuses is reported but exceedingly uncommon [31]. While idiopathic in majority, endocarditis is a rare cause [32]. Surgery is indicated to prevent rupture [32]. Rupture is often into an adjacent heart chamber with high-out heat failure [33]. Surgery consists of patch closure of the involved sinus. Approach can be from the aorta as well as via the other heart chamber that the fistula opens [30].

6. Aortic dissection

Acute aortic dissection is a high-risk aortic catastrophe which occurs in 5–30/1,000,000 patient annually [37]. Almost 1/5th die before reaching the emergency [38]. The initiating factor is often uncontrolled hypertension. Patients may have an intra-mural hematoma prior to developing dissection.

Aortic dissection is classified according to the time after the start of symptoms, being acute if the time frame between the onset of symptoms and presentation is less than 14 days, and chronic if this period is more than 14 days [34]. Anatomical classification is based on the location and extension of the primary tear (**Figure 2**). Dr. DeBakey and colleagues [35] described a method of classification that differentiates the aortic segments involved into: Type I, when the dissections is involving all the aortic segments, while Type II, when the dissection is confined to the ascending aorta, while Type III, when the dissection process is affecting the descending

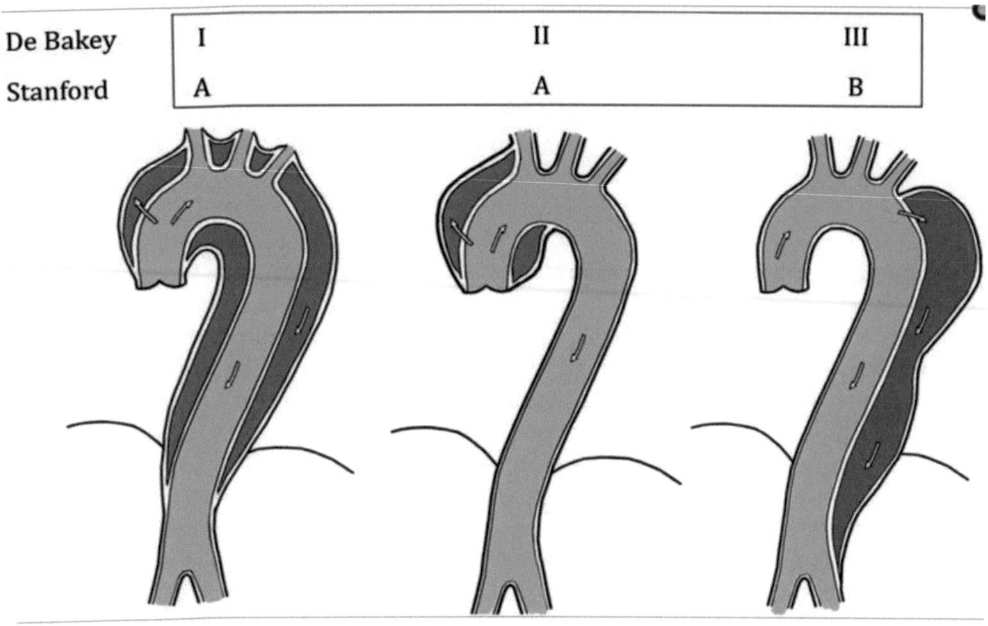

Figure 2.
The anatomical classification of aortic dissection according to the location of the primary tear and the extent of the aortic segment involved are illustrated [36].

thoracic aorta. A more functional classification was introduced by the Stanford University; type A if the dissection involves the ascending aorta, type B if it does not [37].

The devastating complications that may occur with aortic dissection including organ malperfusion syndromes, acute aortic regurgitation, pericardial tamponade and stroke [38]. Surgery is currently the gold standard for acute care of type A aortic dissection [38].

7. Bentall procedure

Bentall and de Bono described their technique of aortic root replacement with a synthetic tube graft and contained prosthetic valve [39]. The coronary ostia were implanted in an end to side fashion without coronary mobilization [39]. Bleeding and pseudo-aneurysms were important complications with their procedure [40]. The present method of coronary mobilization and anastomosis was introduced by Nicholas Kouchoukas [14].

Use of improved graft substitutes and local hemostatic agents have made this procedure safer [41]. Results are good in centers performing these procedures in high volume [40].

The Bentall procedure in younger patients is often performed with a mechanical valve conduit. Appropriate anti-coagulation is important to maintain event-free survival [42]. A recent meta-analysis of 7600 [42] patients who had a mechanical valve conduit reported reoperation rates of Bentall procedure using mechanical valve conduits that the annual linearized rate of occurrence of aortic root re-operation 0.45% (0.039–0.59%). Late mortality was 2.02% (1.77–2.31%) and for hemorrhage was 0.64% (0.47–0.87%) During a mean follow up of 6 years.

However, in older patients, or those who refuse/have contraindications for anti-coagulation, a biologic valve substitute can be used [43]. Gaudino and colleagues demonstrated in a propensity matched cohorts that included patients who underwent aortic root replacement utilizing mechanical valved conduit versus biological valved conduit versus valve sparing procedure that the type of procedure did not influence early or late outcome, however rate of aortic re-operation was 0, 2.4, 7.3% at 5 years for mechanical, biological valved conduits and valve sparing procedure, respectively [43].

8. Aortic root replacement with cryopreserved homograft

Aortic root replacement with cryopreserved homograft tissue is often used for patients with an infected aortic root [44]. The structure of the homograft that includes the muscular part of the left ventricular outflow tract, the anterior mitral leaflet and the aorto-mitral continuity; these provide additional tissue to fill gaps created by aggressive debridement while treating endocarditis [44, 45]. Homograft provide excellent hemodynamics and do not need anti-coagulation. Reports demonstrate improved left ventricular mass regression and ejection fraction after homograft root replacement [46]. However, we would caution their use in young patients. Valve degeneration and subsequent need for re-operation is often inversely proportional to age at implant [44] (**Figure 3**).

We feel that appropriate debridement rather than prosthesis selection determines outcome in patients with aortic root abscess. Jassar et al. reported similar rates of reinfection and reoperation in 134 patients who had aortic root replacement using either cryopreserved homograft, biological or mechanical valved conduits [47].

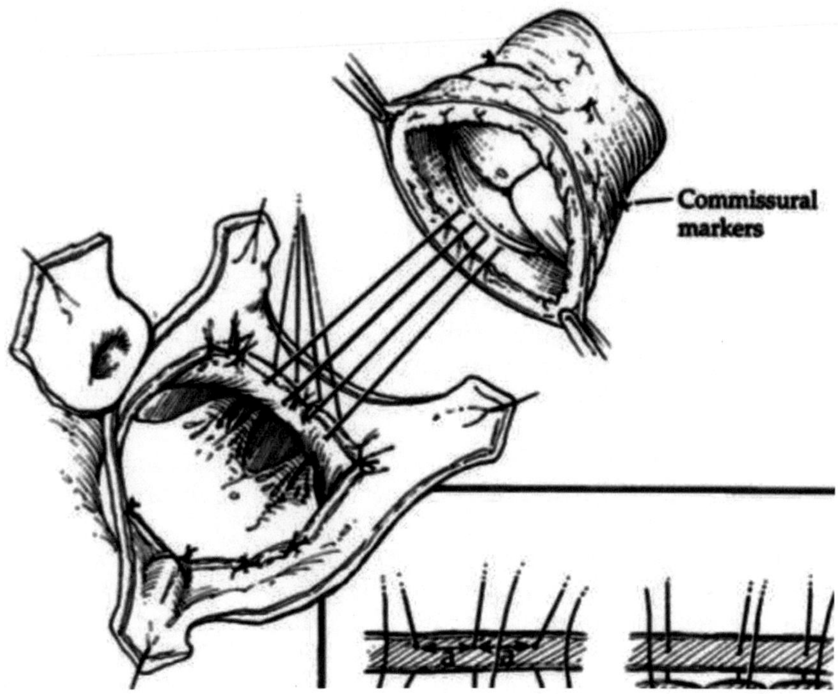

Figure 3.
The insertion of cryopreserved aortic homograft is indicated [48].

DOI: http://dx.doi.org/10.5772/intechopen.86034

9. Aortic root replacement using stentless xenograft

Stent-less valve conduit (Freestyle™ valve conduit, Medtronic Corporation, Minnesota, USA) are commercially easily available when compared to homograft tissue. Thus, in recent years, they are the prosthesis of choice for aortic root replacement in the elderly or those with an infective etiology [49]. Hemodynamics match those of homograft, especially in patients with a small aortic root [50]. The sinus structure of these valves mirrors the native aortic root; an additional benefit when compared to a stented valve conduit [49]. However, unlike stented bio-prostheses, the mechanism of failure of these valves is often leaflet tears [51]. These can occur suddenly leading to acute aortic regurgitation and left heart failure. LeMaire and colleagues demonstrated in 132 patients who had porcine bioroot replacement that there was no structural valve dysfunction in any case during the 5 year follow up period [52] (**Figure 4**).

Here are the relevant steps that we use for our root replacement procedures. These steps remain the same irrespective of the type of prosthesis (mechanical valved-conduit or bioprosthesis):

1. We routinely cannulate the right axillary artery for arterial access in cardiopulmonary bypass in all patients with ascending aortic involvement with aneurysmal disease and certainly in all patients with aortic dissection. Our preferred method is direct cannulation of the axillary artery with a straight cannula (usually 18 or 20Fr); otherwise, an 8 mm vascular graft anastomosed in end-to-side manner to the vessel is used.

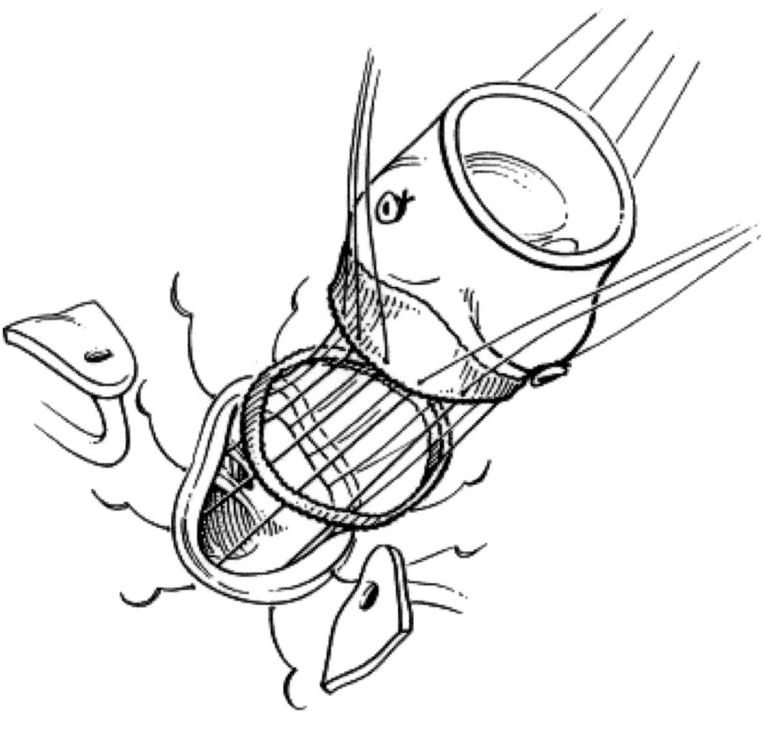

Figure 4.
The free style porcine bioprosthesis with re-implantation of the coronary buttons is demonstrated [53].

2. Upon median sternotomy, pericardium is opened and suspended. Ascending aorta is prepared depending on distal extend of aortic intervention. If feasible, ascending aorta is freed of attachments from the right PA posteriorly and main PA to on the left and taken with an umbilical tape which facilitates further manipulations of the ascending aorta. During this step, it is important to stay close to the aortic wall to avoid injury to the pulmonary artery. For primary aortic root replacement, it is almost always possible to identify and follow such connective tissue plane between the aorta and the pulmonary artery. For a redo operation, it is more difficult and carries some serious risks. We prefer to use cautery dissection rather than scissors or blunt dissection as we feel this technique reduces postoperative bleeding. Small arterial and venous branches are often present between the aorta and pulmonary artery, particularly as one proceeds with dissection more proximally. These are divided between clips. This initial dissection is preferably done prior to full heparinization.

3. Once the ascending aorta is mostly free of attachments and likely looped with an atraumatic tape, we give IV Heparin and cannulate aorta or the right axillary artery and right atrium for cardiopulmonary bypass. We always use retrograde cardioplegia delivered into the coronary sinus and use either a PA or an LV vent inserted via the right superior pulmonary vein.

4. Once aorta is cross-clamped and heart is arrested with a combination of antegrade and retrograde cardioplegia, the aorta is transected in mid portion. Clear identification of the ostium of the right coronary artery (RCA) is required, so that the initial cut through the ascending aorta is placed far enough away from the RCA ostium. It is also important to divide ascending aorta in a way that there is at least a couple of centimeters of the aortic wall above the ostium of the left main coronary artery (LMCA).

5. At this stage we place 4–0 silk stay sutures at the tips of the aortic valve commissures. Aortic valve is then excised, annulus is sized. When a Freestyle valve conduit is used, there is no need to have a cylinder-shaped sizer pass into the LV through the annulus as the prosthetic valve will be fixed in the supra annular position. As such, a larger prosthetic valve can be used. Sizing for a mechanical valve conduit has to be done according to the manufacturer recommendations as most of the mechanical valves are designed for an intra-annular position.

6. At this stage, additional dissection is carried out between the aortic root and pulmonary artery and RVOT. Unlike for a valve sparing aortic root replacement with root re-implantation, this dissection for a Bentall operation is limited to clearing the space for a safe fashioning of the coronary buttons, particularly, for the LMCA. There is no need to dissect deep between the aortic root and the RVOT to expose the aortic annulus from the outside.

7. Preparation of the coronary buttons is similar for any aortic root replacement operation. Normally, we start with the left coronary button. Here are the critical points and pitfalls:

    - Prior to cutting the button out of the corresponding sinus, we recommend marking up the "12 o'clock" point—the top of the button is marked with marker pen or a prolene stitch. This would allow for a precise orientation of the button when re-implanted into a sinus of the valve conduit. Tension or kinking or rotation of the re-implanted button may result in coronary ischemia and create a serious problem at the conclusion of the operation;

- Once the top of the button is marked, we start with cutting the left coronary sinus from the top of the commissure between the left and non-coronary cusps down towards the annulus of the left sinus. Most of the time, the actual opening of the LMCA is kept in the middle of the button on all four aspects of it. In larger root aneurysms, there is occasionally too much tissue in the sinus, so attention should be paid to the size of the button 0.5–1.0 cm off of the edge of the ostium of the LMCA is usually enough for a safe button re-implantation;
- The initial cut has to keep ~5–7 mm of the sinus tissue in place, so as we come down along the commissure, the tip of the scissors is turned away from the annulus and the cut is curved around the lower edge of the coronary artery ostium;
- Next, we start the cut from the top of the commissure between the left and right sinuses. It is critical to fully understand the course of the LMCA to avoid injury to it in case of intramural passing in the aortic wall. Large coronary probe can be placed in the lumen to check the direction of the LMCA. The cut is then curved away from the annulus leaving the same 5–7 mm of the sinus tissue in place and completing a "button" by connecting with incision made from the other direction.
- Great care has to be taken here as to not apply any excessive pulling on any portion of the button while making the cuts as this can lead to distortion and asymmetric fashioning of the button making safe re-implantation difficult;
- Once the LMCA button is fashioned out, the connective tissue and fat between the lower edge of the button and rim of the sinus remnant and the annulus is divided with cautery to provide just enough mobility for the coronary button to facilitate re-implanting process;
- Preparation of the RCA button follows the same general principles as described for the LMCA button—marking the top to maintain orientation, avoiding excessive pulling while fashioning the button, maintaining enough sinus tissue on the button itself as well as on the annulus.

8. After both buttons are prepared, inflow suture line is created. For a mechanical prosthesis, we use 2–0 pledgeted stitches with the pledgets placed in a suppraannular position. It is important to ensure that the pledgets are lined next to each other without much gap as this will ensure hemostasis. Some use a secondary continuous prolene layer to seal this anastomosis. With Freestyle bioprosthesis, we use simple 2–0 interrupted stitches. A pericardial strip is then gently placed between the loops prior to knotting. The pericardial strip acts as a gusset and also provides additional hemostasis to this layer.

9. Additional important point has to be made for cases when Freestyle conduit is used. Orientation of the valve is of critical importance prior to drawing inflow sutures through the valve. We recommend rotating the valve 120°clockwise from its natural orientation, so that a non-coronary sinus of the valve would now become a left coronary sinus into which LMCA is re-implanted. Such rotation will make left coronary sinus of the valve a new right sinus into which RCA button will be re-implanted. The right button of the Freestyle remains unused and has to be over sawn with 4–0 or 5–0 pledgeted sutures.

10. Once an opening in the new left sinus is made with coronary punch, the coronary button is anastomosed using 5–0 prolene. We use a technique of

plicating the wall of the coronary button. A second layer is then used to ensure further hemostasis. Re-implantation of the right button is performed in a similar fashion. Once the aortic root is replaced and buttons re-implanted, we use local hemostatic glue to provide further sealing of needle holes.

11. Then depending upon the extent of aortic dilatation, the ascending aorta is replaced and attached to the proximal neo-root.

12. Once the patient is off cardiopulmonary bypass, the right axillary artery is carefully repaired between hemostatic clamps. A good Doppler signal is essential after repair.

13. It is important to ensure absolute hemostasis in the operating room prior to transferring the patient to the intensive care unit.

10. Valve sparing aortic root replacement

Sparing the patient's native aortic valve while replacing the aortic root is an alternative option in selected patients [54]. This naturally avoids need for anti-coagulation [9]. After an initial pre-operative trans-esophageal echocardiogram, the valve leaflets should be examined prior to proceeding with valve-sparing approach. Leaflet quality is fundamental to event-free survival in these patients.

10.1 Aortic re-implantation technique

David and Feindel [9] recommend a technique of securing the aortic valve leaflets without the rigid synthetic graft. This technique prevents future annular dilatation. Dr. David et al. report excellent valve competence among 146 Marfan's syndrome patients with valve-sparing aortic root replacement with their technique [55] (**Figure 5**).

All preparatory steps for re-implantation procedure are similar as described above. Below are the critical steps unique for the re-implantation:

- Once coronary buttons are prepared as described above, aortic annulus has to be dissected out so that on all sinuses the annulus can be exposed for precise placement of the sub-annular sutures. We use cautery at low settings to perform this dissection. The most difficult part of this step is to separate the root and the annulus from the RVOT. There is always a connective tissue plane between these structures which allows safe dissection down to the annulus;

- Sizing of the annulus can be done by many previously described methods. We prefer to follow a simple rule that most of the male with BSA of ~2.0–2.2 m^2 should have annulus of 23–25 mm, and so 3–5 mm larger diameter of the vascular graft would be chosen (most commonly, 28 or 30 mm). For a smaller female patient with a BSA of 1.8–2.0 m^2 an annular diameter is 21–23 mm and accordingly 26–28 mm grafts are usually appropriate;

- We prefer "Valsalva" grafts (Vascutek) which we trim on the inflow side leaving 2–3 mm (a couple of rings) of the grafts for the sub-annular sutures to be drawn through;

- We then place sub-annular 2–0 ticron sutures with small pledgetes 2–3 mm below the annulus in the following order: the nadir of the non-coronary sinus; the

a

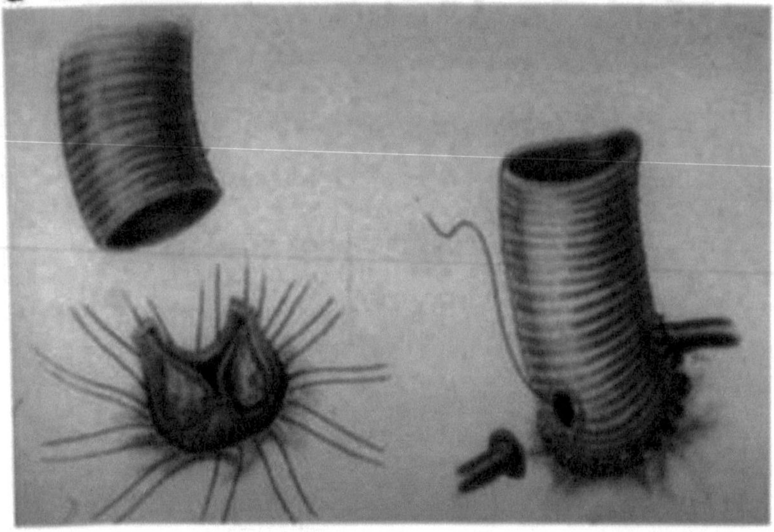

b

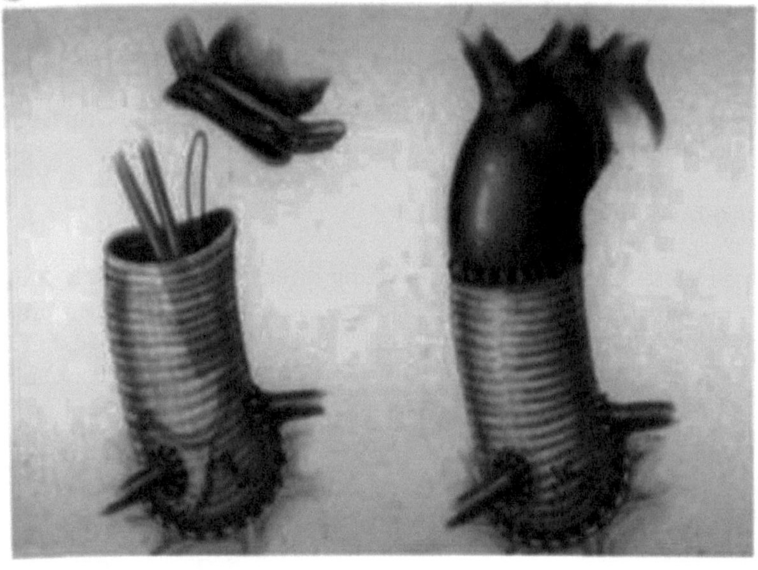

Figure 5.
The aortic re-implantation technique is illustrated (a). As demonstrated, the entire aortic annulus, aortic valve and a rim of aortic wall are all secured inside the synthetic graft, with re-implantation of the coronary buttons to the new graft (b). The distal part of the synthetic graft is anastomosed to the ascending aorta [9].

left-to-non commissure; the nadir of the left coronary sinus; the nadir of the right coronary sinus; the right to-non commissure (avoiding membranous septum); extra sutures placed between the ones mentioned above can added in between the nadirs and the commissural sutures to a total of 6–9 sutures if needed;

- Inflow edge of the Valsalva graft then marked to assure precise positioning of the sub annular sutures on the vascular graft;

- Sub annular sutures are then drawn through the graft according to the markings;

- In re-implantation procedure, instead of silk stay sutures at the tips of the commissures, we use 4–0 prolene with large needles. These stay sutures are brought inside of the graft at this stage, so that the graft is brought over, seated and fixed over the annulus by tying the sub-annular sutures;

- Prolene sutures from the tips of the commissures are then drawn through the graft at the junction of the horizontal and vertical parts of the Valsalva graft;
- Re-implantation of the aortic root is then started by suturing of the remnant of the coronary sinuses inside of the Valsalva graft. We routinely use double armed 4–0 or 5–0 Prolene and start the suture line just off the bottom of the sinus and proceeding towards the commissure between left and non-coronary sinuses bringing the stich to the top of the commissure on the outside. The other arm of the suture is then brought up the same way to the top of the left and right commissure;
- Similar technique is then used to re-implant the right and finally the left coronary sinuses;
- All three stay sutures are then tied and cut on top of the commissures followed by "working" sutures brought to the top of the corresponding commissures;
- The valve is then checked for AI by filling the root with cold saline;
- Coronary buttons are then re-implanted into corresponding sinuses as described above.

10.2 Aortic remodeling technique

Yacoub developed his technique of creating three longitudinal neo-sinuses [56]. These are sutured to the aorta and then coronary buttons are re-implanted. This method does not protect against annular dilatation [9]. In this technique the

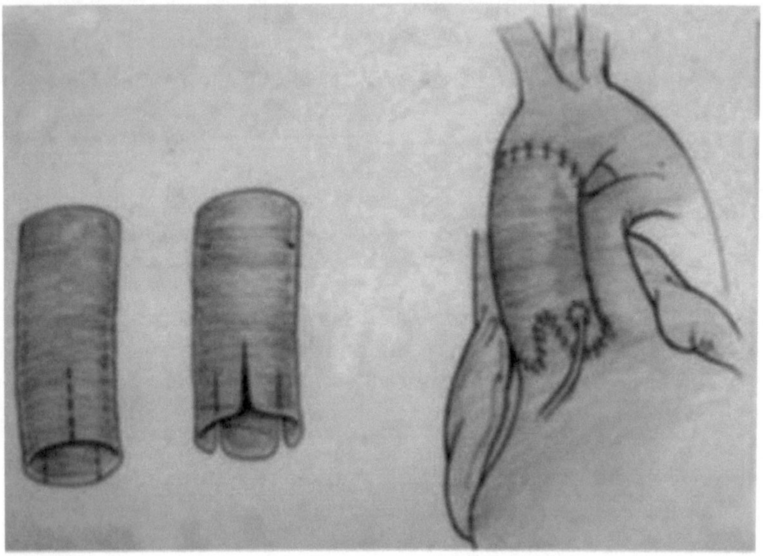

Figure 6.
The aortic remodeling technique is described. As shown, the aortic commissures are sewn to the graft, which is fashioned to form neo sinuses. Then the created tongues are sewn to the rim of the aortic wall. Coronary buttons re-implantation follows, then distal anastomosis between the graft and the ascending aorta is performed [9].

synthetic graft is fashioned into three longitudinal neo sinuses, then after securing the valve commissures to the neo graft, the margins of the neo sinuses are anastomosed to the rim of the aortic wall. Coronary button re-implantation to the neo sinuses follows, and distal anastomosis of the neo graft to the ascending aorta completed the procedure (**Figure 6**).

11. Summary

Aortic root operations reflect complex anatomic relations and physiologic interactions between the left ventricle and components of the aortic root—ventriculo-arterial junction (aortic annulus), sinuses of Valsalva, leaflets of the aortic valve, and sino-tubular junction. Whether a surgeon contemplates classic aortic root replacement with mechanical or tissue valve conduits or any of the valve sparing root reconstructions, close familiarity with the structure and function of the aortic root is necessary. Dreaded complications of such complex procedures (bleeding, most importantly) can be avoided by meticulous surgical technique in combination with intimate knowledge of the anatomical details of the aortic root and surrounding structures.

Disclaimer

The views expressed are those of the authors and do not necessarily reflect the position or policy of the Department of Veteran Affairs or the United States Government.

Author details

Salah E. Altarabsheh[1], Salil V. Deo[2] and Yakov E. Elgudin[2]*

1 Department of Cardiac Surgery, Queen Alia Heart Institute, Amman, Jordan

2 Division of Cardiothoracic Surgery, Louis Stokes Cleveland VA Medical Center, Cleveland, Ohio, USA

*Address all correspondence to: yakov.elgudin@uhhospitals.org

References

[1] Sutton JP 3rd, Ho SY, Anderson RH. The forgotten interleaflet triangles: A review of the surgical anatomy of the aortic valve. The Annals of Thoracic Surgery. 1995;**59**(2):419-427

[2] Anderson RH et al. The myth of the aortic annulus: The anatomy of the subaortic outflow tract. The Annals of Thoracic Surgery. 1991;**52**(3):640-646

[3] Brewer RJ et al. The dynamic aortic root. Its role in aortic valve function. The Journal of Thoracic and Cardiovascular Surgery. 1976;**72**(3):413-417

[4] David TE. An anatomic and physiologic approach to acquired heart disease. 8th Annual Meeting of the European Cardio-thoracic Association, The Hague, Netherlands, September 25-28, 1994. European Journal of Cardio-Thoracic Surgery. 1995;**9**(4):175-180

[5] Underwood MJ et al. The aortic root: Structure, function, and surgical reconstruction. Heart. 2000;**83**(4):376-380

[6] Ho SY. Structure and anatomy of the aortic root. European Journal of Echocardiography. 2009;**10**(1):i3-i10

[7] Charitos EI, Sievers HH. Anatomy of the aortic root: Implications for valve-sparing surgery. Annals Cardiothorac Surgery. 2013;**2**(1):53-56

[8] Thubrikar MJ et al. Stress sharing between the sinus and leaflets of canine aortic valve. The Annals of Thoracic Surgery. 1986;**42**(4):434-440

[9] Feindel CM, David TE. Aortic valve sparing operations: Basic concepts. International Journal of Cardiology. 2004;**97**(Suppl 1):61-66

[10] Becker DG et al. Clinical study of alar anatomy and surgery of the alar base. Archives of Otolaryngology-Head and Neck Surgery. 1997;**123**(8):789-795

[11] Cannata A, Russo CF, Vitali E. Bicuspid aortic valve: About natural history of ascending aorta aneurysms. The Annals of Thoracic Surgery. 2008;**85**(1):362-363

[12] David TE, Maganti M, Armstrong S. Aortic root aneurysm: Principles of repair and long-term follow-up. The Journal of Thoracic and Cardiovascular Surgery. 2010;**140**(6 Suppl):S14-S19; discussion S45-51

[13] Augoustides JG, Plappert T, Bavaria JE. Aortic decision-making in the Loeys-Dietz syndrome: Aortic root aneurysm and a normal-caliber ascending aorta and aortic arch. The Journal of Thoracic and Cardiovascular Surgery. 2009;**138**(2):502-503

[14] Coselli JS. It's time to get to the root of things. The Journal of Thoracic and Cardiovascular Surgery. 2016;**151**(2):291-293

[15] Song HK et al. Long-term implications of emergency versus elective proximal aortic surgery in patients with Marfan syndrome in the genetically triggered thoracic aortic aneurysms and cardiovascular conditions consortium registry. The Journal of Thoracic and Cardiovascular Surgery. 2012;**143**(2):282-286

[16] Loeys BL et al. A syndrome of altered cardiovascular, craniofacial, neurocognitive and skeletal development caused by mutations in TGFBR1 or TGFBR2. Nature Genetics. 2005;**37**(3):275-281

[17] Atzinger CL et al. Cross-sectional and longitudinal assessment of aortic root dilation and valvular anomalies in hypermobile and classic Ehlers-Danlos syndrome. The Journal of Pediatrics. 2011;**158**(5):826-830. e1

[18] Borger MA et al. The American association for thoracic surgery consensus guidelines on bicuspid aortic valve-related aortopathy: Full online-only version. The Journal of Thoracic and Cardiovascular Surgery. 2018;**156**(2):e41-e74

[19] Siu SC, Silversides CK. Bicuspid aortic valve disease. Journal of the American College of Cardiology. 2010;**55**(25):2789-2800

[20] Bonderman D et al. Mechanisms underlying aortic dilatation in congenital aortic valve malformation. Circulation. 1999;**99**(16):2138-2143

[21] Nistri S et al. Aortic elasticity and size in bicuspid aortic valve syndrome. European Heart Journal. 2008;**29**(4):472-479

[22] Ostberg G. An arteritis with special reference to polymyalgia arteritica. Acta Pathologica et Microbiologica Scandinavica. Supplement. 1973;**237**(Suppl 237):1-59

[23] Kerr GS et al. Takayasu arteritis. Annals of Internal Medicine. 1994;**120**(11):919-929

[24] Robinson WP 3rd et al. Fulminant development of mega-aorta due to Takayasu's arteritis: Case report and review of the literature. Vascular. 2005;**13**(3):178-183

[25] Song MH et al. Aortic root aneurysm in Takayasu arteritis syndrome: Exploration in active phase and repair in inactive phase. The Journal of Thoracic and Cardiovascular Surgery. 2008;**136**(4):1084-1085

[26] Yuan SM, Jing H. Cystic medial necrosis: Pathological findings and clinical implications. Revista Brasileira de Cirurgia Cardiovascular. 2011;**26**(1):107-115

[27] Borger MA et al. The American Association for Thoracic Surgery consensus guidelines on bicuspid aortic valve-related aortopathy: Executive summary. The Journal of Thoracic and Cardiovascular Surgery. 2018;**156**(2):473-480

[28] Gott VL et al. Replacement of the aortic root in patients with Marfan's syndrome. The New England Journal of Medicine. 1999;**340**(17):1307-1313

[29] Joint Task Force on the Management of Valvular Heart Disease of the European Society of Cardiology (ESC) et al. Guidelines on the management of valvular heart disease (version 2012). European Heart Journal. 2012;**33**(19):2451-2496

[30] Altarabsheh SE et al. Unruptured sinus of valsalva aneurysm involving all three sinuses. The Annals of Thoracic Surgery. 2011;**91**(2):e26-e27

[31] Yan F et al. Surgery for sinus of valsalva aneurysm: 27-year experience with 100 patients. Asian Cardiovascular & Thoracic Annals. 2008;**16**(5):361-365

[32] Bhat PS et al. Aneurysm of all 3 sinuses of valsalva causing coronary insufficiency. Asian Cardiovascular & Thoracic Annals. 2009;**17**(6):637-639

[33] Lijoi A et al. Unruptured aneurysm of the left sinus of valsalva causing coronary insufficiency: Case report and review of the literature. Texas Heart Institute Journal. 2002;**29**(1):40-44

[34] Atkins MD Jr, Black JH 3rd, Cambria RP. Aortic dissection:

Perspectives in the era of stent-graft repair. Journal of Vascular Surgery. 2006;**43**(Suppl A):30A-43A

[35] Debakey ME et al. Surgical management of dissecting aneurysms of the aorta. The Journal of Thoracic and Cardiovascular Surgery. 1965;**49**:130-149

[36] Erbel R et al. Diagnosis and management of aortic dissection. European Heart Journal. 2001;**22**(18):1642-1681

[37] Daily PO et al. Management of acute aortic dissections. The Annals of Thoracic Surgery. 1970;**10**(3):237-247

[38] Gawinecka J, Schonrath F, von Eckardstein A. Acute aortic dissection: Pathogenesis, risk factors and diagnosis. Swiss Medical Weekly. 2017;**147**:w14489

[39] Bentall H, De Bono A. A technique for complete replacement of the ascending aorta. Thorax. 1968;**23**(4):338-339

[40] Kirsch EW et al. Aortic root replacement after previous surgical intervention on the aortic valve, aortic root, or ascending aorta. The Journal of Thoracic and Cardiovascular Surgery. 2006;**131**(3):601-608

[41] Loisance D. Simplification of the Bentall procedure with surgical and biological innovations. European Journal of Cardio-Thoracic Surgery. 1994;**8**(11):613-615

[42] Mookhoek A et al. Bentall procedure: A systematic review and meta-analysis. The Annals of Thoracic Surgery. 2016;**101**(5):1684-1689

[43] Gaudino M et al. Contemporary outcomes of surgery for aortic root aneurysms: A propensity-matched comparison of valve-sparing and composite valve graft replacement. The Journal of Thoracic and Cardiovascular Surgery. 2015;**150**(5):1120-1129.e1

[44] Sultan I et al. Aortic root replacement with cryopreserved homograft for infective endocarditis in the modern north American opioid epidemic. The Journal of Thoracic and Cardiovascular Surgery. 2019;**157**(1):45-50

[45] Solari S et al. Over 20 years experience with aortic homograft in aortic valve replacement during acute infective endocarditis. European Journal of Cardio-Thoracic Surgery. 2016;**50**(6):1158-1164

[46] Kunadian B et al. Meta-analysis of valve hemodynamics and left ventricular mass regression for stentless versus stented aortic valves. The Annals of Thoracic Surgery. 2007;**84**(1):73-78

[47] Jassar AS et al. Graft selection for aortic root replacement in complex active endocarditis: Does it matter? The Annals of Thoracic Surgery. 2012;**93**(2):480-487

[48] Northrup WF 3rd, Kshettry VR. Implantation technique of aortic homograft root: Emphasis on matching the host root to the graft. The Annals of Thoracic Surgery. 1998;**66**(1):280-284

[49] Tavakoli R et al. Full-root aortic valve replacement with stentless xenograft achieves superior regression of left ventricular hypertrophy compared to pericardial stented aortic valves. Journal of Cardiothoracic Surgery. 2015;**10**:15

[50] Kunihara T et al. Root replacement using stentless valves in the small aortic root: A propensity score analysis. The Annals of Thoracic Surgery. 2006;**82**(4):1379-1384

[51] Grande KJ et al. Porcine aortic leaflet arrangement may contribute

to clinical xenograft failure. ASAIO Journal. 1993;**39**(4):918-922

[52] LeMaire SA et al. Aortic root replacement with stentless porcine xenografts: Early and late outcomes in 132 patients. The Annals of Thoracic Surgery. 2009;**87**(2):503-512; discussion 512-3

[53] Kon ND et al. Aortic root replacement with the freestyle stentless porcine aortic root bioprosthesis. The Annals of Thoracic Surgery. 1999;**67**(6):1609-1615; discussion 1615-6

[54] Ouzounian M et al. Valve-sparing root replacement compared with composite valve graft procedures in patients with aortic root dilation. Journal of the American College of Cardiology. 2016;**68**(17):1838-1847

[55] David TE et al. Outcomes of aortic valve-sparing operations in Marfan syndrome. Journal of the American College of Cardiology. 2015;**66**(13):1445-1453

[56] Sarsam MA, Yacoub M. Remodeling of the aortic valve anulus. The Journal of Thoracic and Cardiovascular Surgery. 1993;**105**(3):435-438

Chapter 5

Minimally Invasive Right Anterior Mini-Thoracotomy Aortic Valve Replacement

Imran Khan, Julian A. Smith and Naresh Trehan

Abstract

Since the emergence of small skin incision aortic valve surgery in the late 1990s, minimally invasive aortic valve replacement has now become a viable alternative to standard full sternotomy. The spectrum includes (a) upper hemi sternotomy (T or J shaped), (b) lower partial sternotomy, and (c) right anterior mini-thoracotomy. Potential advantages include a cosmetically appealing scar, decreased post-operative pain and bleeding, shorter ventilation time and hospital stay, and early return to active life. The operative challenges include restricted view and access to the operative field, longer aortic cross-clamp time, and cardiopulmonary bypass time. This necessitates detailed pre-operative imaging, correct selection and assessment of patients, and good communication with perfusionists and anesthetists regarding the plan of each surgery, with a solid back-up plan in case conversion to full sternotomy is required intra-operatively. In recent times, the use of suture less valves and rapid deployment bio prosthesis has dramatically reduced operative time. Here, we describe the work-up, selection criteria, key steps, and potential pitfalls of the right anterior mini-thoracotomy approach for aortic valve replacement.

Keywords: minimally invasive aortic valve replacement, suture less valve, rapid deployment bio prosthesis, work-up, pitfalls, imaging

1. Introduction

Conventional full median sternotomy aortic valve replacement (AVR) has remained the standard approach to AVR for many years. In-hospital mortality of 2.3% for isolated conventional AVR (22,107 patients) has been reported in German Aortic Valve Registry [1]. Despite these excellent results, full sternotomy incision has been criticized for its length, postoperative pain and possible complications including sternal wound dehiscence, which dramatically increase the morbidity of the procedure [2].

The introduction of minimally invasive aortic valve surgery began in the last decade of twentieth century. The first minimally invasive AVR was performed by Cosgrove and Sabik in 1996 using a parasternal approach [3]. Bennetti et al. used the right thoracotomy approach in 1997 [4]. In 1998, Gundry et al. [5] reported a partial upper mini sternotomy approach in both adult valve and congenital procedures. Minimally invasive aortic valve surgery has recently moved from simple modifications of conventional steps to totally endoscopic aortic valve replacement (TEAVR) [6].

IntechOpen

Although results of many retrospective and prospective studies behold a bright future for this approach, the prevalence of minimally invasive aortic valve replacement (MIAVR) has not met potential expectations: 29% of AVRs are done minimally invasive in Germany [7] and 12% in the UK [8]. Kaneko et al. [9] reported that 12% patients had hemi sternotomy AVR and 3.6% patients were operated via an anterior mini-thoracotomy approach in the USA.

A possibly long learning curve and complexity of the procedure may dissuade the widespread uptake of MIAVR. In an era of trans-catheter aortic valve implantation (TAVI) [10], sufficient motivation should be present for cardiac surgeons to adopt MIAVR in majority of patients, especially considering the recent promising results [11].

2. Why cardiac surgeons should adopt minimally invasive aortic valve surgery?

Minimally invasive cardiac surgery is a thought process that aims to minimize the extent of surgical invasiveness [12]. The American Heart Association (2008) defined it as "a small chest wall incision that does not include the conventional full sternotomy" [13]. The STS database defines minimally invasive cardiac surgery as "any procedure not performed with full sternotomy and cardiopulmonary bypass (CPB) support" [14]. The AHA definition is more realistic in the sense that an open heart surgery procedure is more likely to be conducted with cardiopulmonary bypass support. Based on the current STS definition, only TAVI can be included.

Potential advantages of MIAVR are:

a. Cosmesis and wound complications: Improved cosmesis and esthetic scar is the unquestionable benefit of MIAVR. Although superficial wound infections have been reported [15], avoiding a full sternotomy leads to complete avoidance of deep sternal wound infection and risk of sternal non-union. Patients are discharged from ICU and hospital earlier and they return to an active work life earlier compared to full sternotomy AVR [16].

b. Post-operative bleeding and blood transfusions: The need for blood transfusion was reported to be reduced in patients undergoing MIVAR compared to full sternotomy AVR (36 vs. 52.4%, <0.001) [17]. Burdett et al. [18] showed that MIAVR patients had significantly less post-operative blood loss (232 vs. 513 ml, $p = 0.00021$) and were less likely to require blood products (fresh frozen plasma and platelets) (24 vs. 36%, $p = 0.042$).

c. Post-operative pain: Randomized control trials (RCTs) [19] and meta-analysis [20] have shown reduced pain scores with MIAVR. Limited spreading and retraction of the chest wall minimizes the disruption of the costo-chondral and costo vertebral joints. It leads to decreased use of narcotic analgesia in the post-operative period and early ambulation, leading to a more rapid return to an active work life.

d. Ventilation time: Stolinski et al. [21] reported ventilation time of 9.7 +/ 5.9 h after AVR and 7.2 +/ 3.2 h after ART-AVR ($p < 0.001$). Pulmonary function test results were lower in conventional AVR than RAMT-AVR ($p = 0.001$) for FEV1, vital capacity, total lung capacity. Phan et al. [17] also showed a reduction in ventilation time of more than 4 h with MIAVR.

e. Cost-benefit analysis: Due to reduced ventilation time, blood transfusion requirements, shorter ICU and hospital stay, total hospital costs were lower in minimally AVR group ($36,348 vs. $38,239, $p = 0.02$) [22].

f. Mortality: Joseph Lamelas [23] reported a 30-day mortality of 1.63% in 857 isolated MIAVR. Glauber et al. [11] reported in-hospital mortality of 1.5% in 593 patients. At 31.5 months mean follow up time, 94.8% survival was observed.

3. Patient selection

Optimum patient selection is essential for MIAVR. The factors to be taken into consideration include individual surgeon preference and skill sets, the patient's anatomical factors and comorbidities. The commitment and experience of the entire surgical team including anesthetists and perfusionists plays a critical role in the successful outcome.

3.1 Indications

Patients presenting with severe and/or symptomatic aortic valve stenosis or insufficiency requiring an isolated AVR are potential candidates for MIAVR.

3.2 Contraindications

1. Unfavorable chest anatomy: Exposure and operative access to the ascending aorta and aortic valve are compromised in severe chest wall deformities and dislocation of heart and great vessels (e.g., pectus excavatum).

2. Previous thoracic surgery: Patients with previous thoracic surgery—pleurodesis, lobectomy, and pneumonectomy have compromised anatomical exposure and access to the operative field. Such a situation also increases the risks [24] of perioperative complications—bleeding, air leak, conversation to full sternotomy.

3. Calcified ascending aorta: Assessment of a safe area for arterial cannulation and applying the aortic cross clamp requires optimum exposure. Control of bleeding from a calcified aorta—cannulation site, aortotomy—is potentially challenging with limited exposure.

4. Re-operation: Previous cardiac surgery is not an absolute contraindication to MIAVR. It may be a suitable option after previous valvular surgery. However, previous CABG is a contraindication due to risk of damaging patient's bypass grafts and also of inadequate myocardial protection. With full sternotomy, myocardial protection through retrograde cardioplegia, topical cooling and temporary occlusion of patent LIMA during cardioplegic arrest is possible.

5. Small aortic root (<19 mm) or aneurysmal dilation of aorta/sinuses: It may necessitate a concomitant aortic root enlargement and/or aortic root replacement procedure which is better achieved through full sternotomy.

6. Severe left ventricular dysfunction: Patients with an ejection fraction <30%, dilated left ventricles are more prone to intra-operative hemodynamic instability and arrhythmias. These situations can be better managed through full sternotomy.

7. Previous radiotherapy or pericarditis: These lead to intra thoracic and pericardial adhesions making dissection difficult. Temporary epicardial pacing wires may not be placed effectively requiring trans-venous pacing.

3.3 Clinical assessment

Pre-operative physical examination is a mandatory step in the work up and appropriate selection of patients. Important considerations are:

a. Previous incisions in the chest and groin: These indicate adhesions and distortion of anatomy in the area of dissection. If there are adhesions around right atrium, femoral venous cannulation is a good alternative. It allows for increased exposure of aortic root and ascending aorta.

b. Increased chest rigidity: Partial retraction of sternum in upper hemi-sternotomy (UHS) or ribs in anterior right mini-thoracotomy (ART) is required for exposure. Increased chest rigidity due to previous chest surgery, chest trauma or ankylosing spondylitis can compromise the retraction required for exposure. Very muscular and, more commonly in young patients, slightly stiff chest walls can be encountered. Costochondral cartilages can be transected in patients with narrow intercostal spaces. Such a step helps to increase exposure. These can be sutured back into position at the end of procedure.

c. Chest wall deformity: Pectus excavatum is the most common chest wall deformity [25]. It displaces heart to the left. Patients with moderate or severe pectus excavatum with Haller index >3.2 are contraindicated.

d. Morbid obesity: In obese patients the heart is more cranially displaced, due to excess fat in abdomen. It improves the exposure and access to ascending aorta. But there is also increased difficulty in getting into chest cavity due to abundant subcutaneous and mediastinal fat.

e. Height: In very tall patients (>185 cm), peripheral venous cannula may not reach the superior vena cava leading to insufficient venous drainage and distention of right atrium/ventricle. Insertion of another venous cannula into superior vena cava and connecting it to venous line through Y-connector can help improve the venous drainage. However, the heart is more caudally placed in very tall patients, impacting the distance to be negotiated to reach the aortic valve.

4. Pre-operative investigations

1. Chest X-ray: It helps to (a) identify acute and chronic lung pathology, (b) assess basic thoracic anatomy and (c) To note generally that aortic valve is in close relation to 4th intercostal space.

2. ECG: Pre-operative conduction disorders are an independent risk factor for permanent pacemaker insertion [26]. Use of rapid deployment or suture less bio prosthesis increases the risk of complete atrioventricular block. The possible reason could be increased pressure on aortic annulus and left ventricular outflow tract (LVOT) and then on the conduction tissue.

3. Echocardiography: It is the gold standard to assess the aortic valve pathology. Size of the aortic annulus, gradients across the aortic valve, bicuspid or tricuspid aortic valve, and left ventricle ejection fraction are all the important information to be gathered prior to surgery.

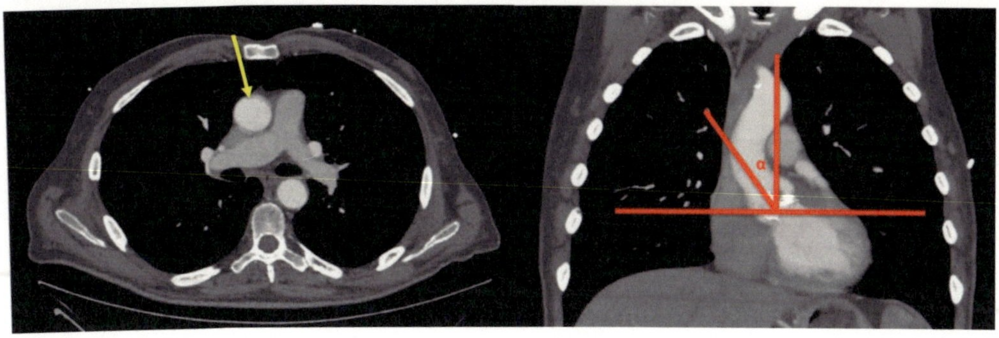

Figure 1.
At the level of the main pulmonary artery, the ascending aorta is rightward (more than one half located on the right in respect to the right sternal border). The distance from the ascending aorta to the sternum does not exceed 10 cm.

4. CT-scan: Pre-operative non-contrast axial CT scan is mandatory before MIAVR through a right anterior mini-thoracotomy (RAMT) approach, in contrast to mini-sternotomy (MS) approach. Patients are suitable for RAMT-MIAVR only if the following criteria are met: (a) At the level of main pulmonary artery, the ascending aorta is rightward (more than one half located on the right in respect to the right sternal border.) (b) The distance from ascending aorta to sternum does not exceed 10 cm. (c) The alpha angle (angle between angle midline and inclination of ascending aorta) should be >45° (**Figure 1**).

5. Coronary angiography: It is the gold standard investigation for detection of coronary artery anatomy and pathology. Its importance is (a) to detect abnormal coronary anatomy which influences myocardial protection strategies (b) in finding of critical coronary artery lesions which may change an isolated AVR procedure to AVR + CABG. This will change the approach for the procedure required to a full sternotomy.

6. Peripheral femoral Doppler: It is an extremely important investigation to assess the size of femoral vessels especially the femoral artery. Diameter less than 5 mm may not be adequate for femoral arterial cannulation and to maintain adequate flows on cardiopulmonary bypass. Also, it is important to rule out any atherosclerotic plaques in femoral arteries, which can interfere with the passing of a guide wire for femoral cannulation. If so, it may be necessary to change the cannulation site from femoral to central.

5. Surgical techniques

The two most commonly used approaches today are (a) Ministernotomy and (b) Right anterior minithoracotomy (**Figure 2**).

a. Ministernotomy: It is the most common technique in use. A 6–10 cm midline vertical incision, with a partial J sternotomy is made. Murtuza et al. [27] reported superior results in peri-operative mortality, shorter ventilation time, ICU and hospital stay compared to full sternotomy AVR.

b. Right anterior minithoracotomy: It is the second most frequently used approach. Few studies have analyzed this approach. Glauber et al. [28] in their 192 patient series reported 0.7% in-hospital mortality. Compared to mini-sternotomy, right anterior mini-thoracotomy patients had lower post-operative

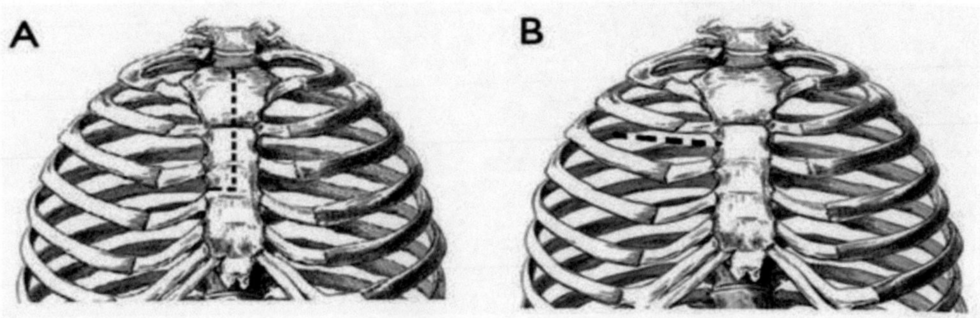

Figure 2.
Minimally invasive incisions: (A) mini sternotomy, (B) right anterior mini thoracotomy.

atrial fibrillation (19.5 vs. 34.2%), shorter ventilation time (median 7 vs. 8 h = 0.003) and a shorter hospital stay (median 5 vs. 6 days) [29].

6. Right anterior mini-thoracotomy approach

We shall now discuss our technique outlining key steps, safeguards and pitfalls.

6.1 Patient positioning and preparation

It is very important to communicate clearly with all team members including anesthetists, perfusionists and theatre nursing staff, the minimally invasive approach planned.

1. Patient is placed supine with a pressure bag inflated below the right shoulder to slightly elevate the right chest.

2. Midline sternotomy incision is marked in case emergency conversion is required intraoperatively. Wide preparation of the chest.

3. Incision is marked in the right 2nd intercostal space for right anterior mini-thoracotomy.

4. Trans-oesophageal echocardiography (TOE) is a mandatory tool to help in placement of femoral venous cannula and retrograde cardioplegia cannula.

5. Defibrillation pads should be attached on the left side of the chest and on the back. Sterile pediatric internal paddles should be available on table, in case external defibrillator pads malfunction.

6. Sternal saw is kept on table, if required in emergency so that precious time is not wasted.

7. Both groins are exposed. It is important to angulate the operation table to optimally expose the groin.

8. Right radial catheter and Swan Ganz catheter is inserted.

9. Left internal jugular vein central line is inserted if central SVC cannulation is planned.

6.2 Chest Approach

1. Chest is opened first as it helps in first hand inspection of pleural cavity and also helps in manual guidance of femoral venous cannula towards superior vena cava.

2. 5–6 cm transverse incision is made over right 2nd intercostal space.

3. Right internal mammary artery and vein are clipped and divided.

4. Inferior rib is transected at the costochondral junction which can be re-approximated with a vicryl suture at the end of the procedure. It increases the operative space and is a much better option than forceful mechanical retraction.

5. Soft tissue retractor and intercostal rib spreader further increase the exposure.

6. Pericardium is opened over right atrium and extended towards the inferior vena cava taking care of the phrenic nerve. Pericardial opening is extended towards the ascending aorta, carefully dissecting the thymic fat. Care is taken not to open the pericardium up to its attachment to aorta, as it can compromise pericardial stay suture placement. Carefully placed pericardial sutures provide exposure of the aorta.

6.3 Cannulation for cardio-pulmonary bypass

About 3–4 cm transverse incision is made above the right inguinal crease. Femoral artery and vein along with branches are dissected and looped with vascular tape. Vascular clamp is placed proximally. Longitudinal incision is made over femoral artery and vein and cannulae are inserted into respective vessels after releasing the vascular clamp. Alternatively, a Seldinger technique may be used for peripheral vessel cannulation (**Figure 3**).

Cannula size is based on the size of the femoral vessels and body surface area. The femoral venous cannula is placed into the SVC under TOE guidance. After femoral decannulation, femoral vessels are repaired with prolene 6-0/7-0.

If peripheral vascular disease is suspected, axillary or central aortic cannulation is performed.

Vacuum assisted venous drainage of 30–70 mmHg as needed may be used to maintain bypass flows and to decompress the right heart. If venous drainage is inadequate, additional central SVC cannulation is required.

6.4 Myocardial protection

Under TOE guidance, a retrograde cardioplegia cannula is inserted through right atrium body/appendage. Its downward retraction facilitates the exposure of the aorta (**Figures 4** and **5**).

A left ventricular vent is passed through right superior pulmonary vein. It is very helpful in unloading the heart and also in deairing the heart while coming off cardiopulmonary bypass.

The aorta is cross clamped using Chitwood clamp through separate incision in the chest wall near the anterior axillary line. Dissection between aorta and pulmonary artery is not required. If bleeding occurs in this area, it is difficult to control.

Antegrade cardioplegia is delivered. If such is not possible due to moderate or severe aortic regurgitation, direct coronary ostial cardioplegia can be given along with retrograde cardioplegia. A CO_2 catheter is placed in the operative field for de airing.

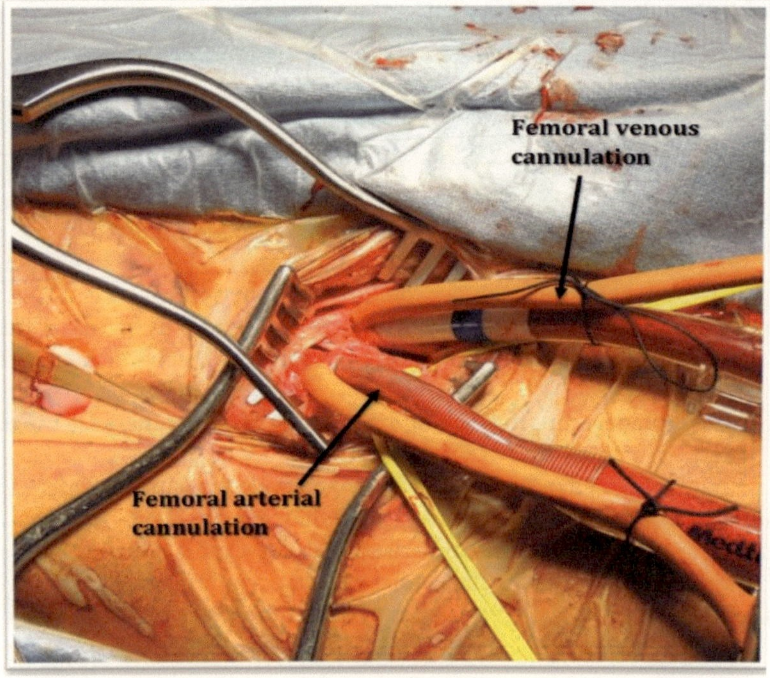

Figure 3.
Peripheral femoral cannulation.

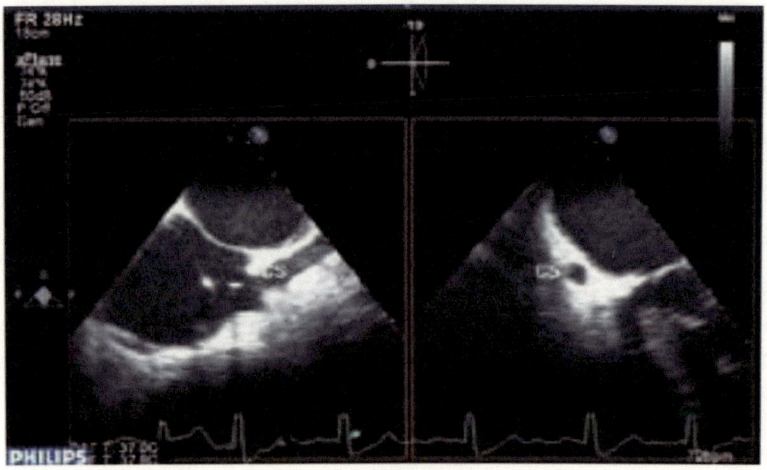

Figure 4.
Retrograde cardioplegia cannula in coronary sinus under TOE guidance.

6.5 Aortotomy

The aortotomy is made at the level of fat pad on aorta. Stay sutures are placed on either edge of the aortotomy for retraction. Resection of valve leaflets, debridement of annulus and valve replacement is done as per standard techniques (**Figures 6** and 7).

Resection and decalcification of a severely stenotic calcified valve is the most difficult step. Using commissural stay sutures and aortic wall retraction sutures significantly improve the exposure. Placing small wet gauze inside the left ventricle

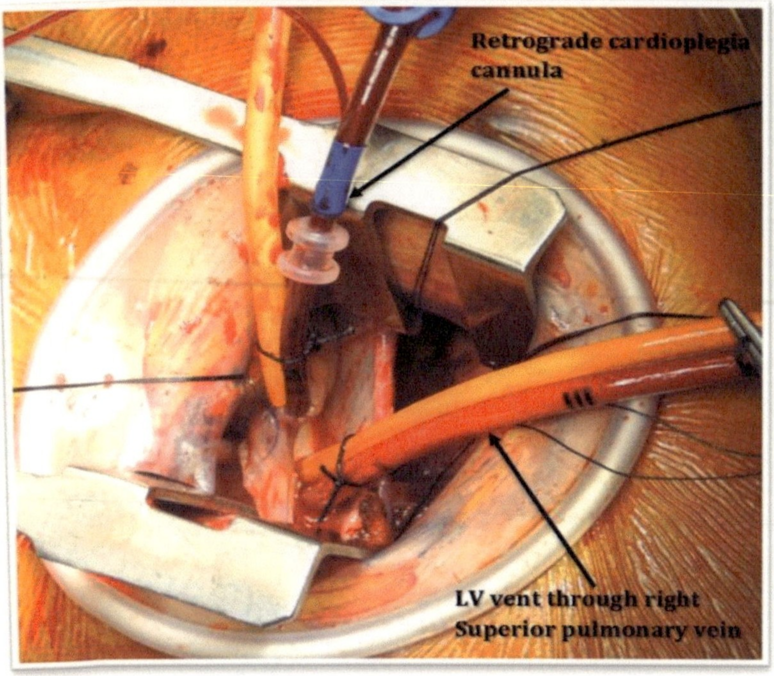

Figure 5.
Retrograde cardioplegia with LV vent in situ.

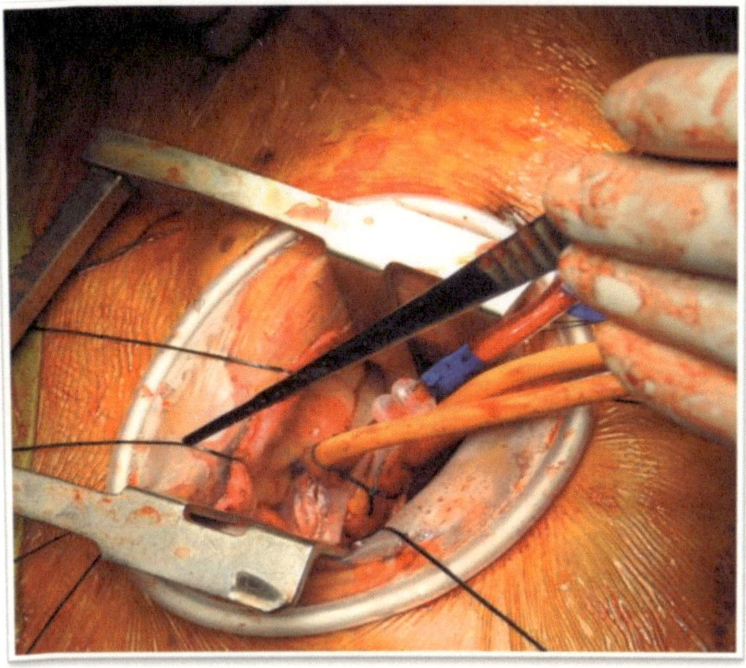

Figure 6.
Aorta cross-clamped with Chitwood clamp through separate skin stab.

while doing decalcification prevents small calcium fragments from getting lost. This wet gauze can be taken out after decalcification has been completed. Similar to the conventional sternotomy approach, decalcification should be followed by thorough saline flushing of the left ventricle (**Figures 8** and **9**).

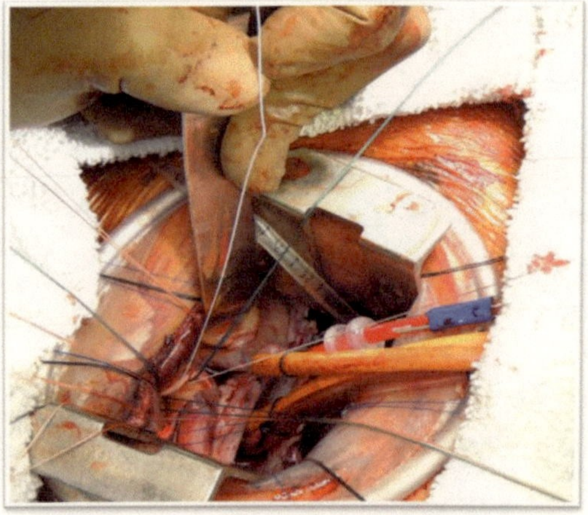

Figure 7.
Aortic valve sutures in place—interrupted pledgeted.

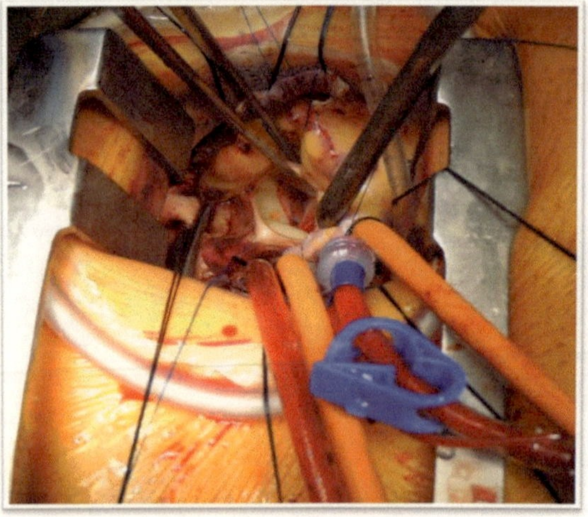

Figure 8.
Aortic valve replaced.

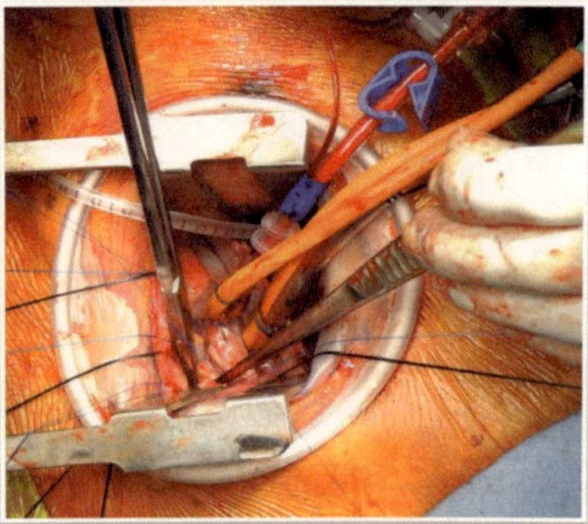

Figure 9.
Aortotomy closure.

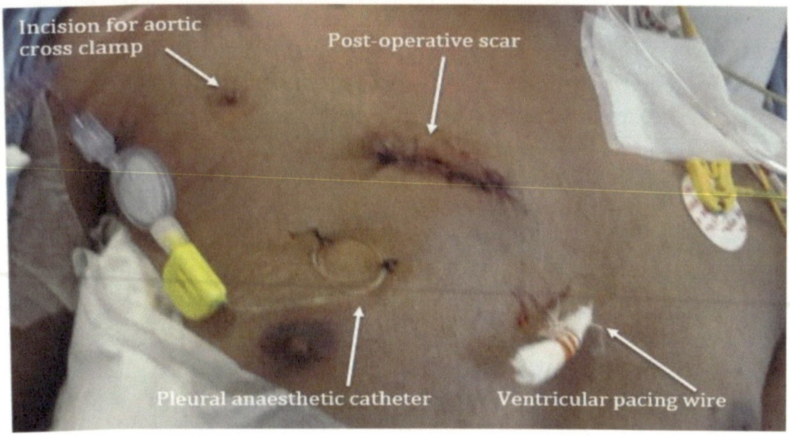

Figure 10.
Post-operative scar.

6.6 Pacemaker wire placement

After aortotomy closure, but before removing the cross clamp, ventricular pacing wire (s) is/are placed on the anterior aspect of the right ventricle. It's extremely difficult to place pacing wires on a beating right ventricle and sometimes, bleeding from the right ventricle can force conversion to sternotomy.

Defibrillation is performed using external pads or pediatric paddles if required.

6.7 Deairing

After aortotomy closure and before the cross clamp is removed, ventilate the lungs and fill the heart and remove the air through the aortic root vent. Insufflating the operative field with carbon dioxide gas helps in deairing. It's important to ventilate the lungs and let the heart eject blood during the reperfusion period. TOE plays a very important role in assessing the effectiveness of deairing maneuvers.

The heart is not manipulated directly for air removal maneuvers. Left-right positioning of patient and external compression of chest wall and forceful shaking of rib retractor may be performed to agitate and disperse air bubbles.

6.8 Weaning from cardio-pulmonary bypass and closure

After appropriate ABG results and optimum rewarming, CPB is gradually discontinued. Femoral venous and arterial cannulas are removed and femoral vessels repaired with Prolene 6-0/7-0.

For pain relief, epidural anesthetic catheter is placed into pleural space and 0.25% bupivacaine is given for 72 h.

Ribs are approximated with vicryl or prolene suture and muscle layers closed in standard fashion (**Figure 10**).

7. Conversion to full sternotomy

Conversion to full sternotomy is a psychological stress for the team and an additional scar on the patient. It occurs in 0.8–8.0% with 3–4% average in most of the series [20]. Possible reasons include inadequate exposure, bleeding from the right ventricle, aortotomy site or right internal mammary, or an inability to defibrillate. A ministernotomy incision can be extended to full sternotomy. With right mini-thoracotomy, incision can be extended to a transverse sternotomy or, alternatively, full sternotomy can be created. It leads to longer bypass times, adding to the morbidity of the procedure [30].

8. Sutureless MIAVR

Encouraging results have been reported with the three different suture less or rapid deployment bio prosthesis [31, 32]. Micelli et al. [33] reported 38 and 40% decrease in cross clamp and CPB time in RAMT group and 43 and 35% decrease in MS group. The operative mortality was 0.7% with a very low incidence of paravalvular leak (1.8%), a frequent complication of TAVI.

Santarpino et al. [34] reported similar improved results with suture less valves, suggesting that suture less MIAVR may become the first line treatment in high risk patients in the spectrum between TAVI and conventional AVR. Randomized controlled trials are required to confirm this.

9. Concerns regarding MIAVR

Although MIAVR has shown consistently good results compared to full sternotomy, there are still areas of concern:

a. MIAVR is associated with longer cross clamp and CPB times, which are known to have adverse impact upon the results. These times assume greater significance in elderly and high-risk patients. However, the use of suture less valves has significantly reduced these times.

b. MIAVR is not very "surgeon friendly" due to being a complex and technically challenging procedure. It has a longer learning curve due to the deeper operative field and limited working space for exposure and implantation of the prosthetic valve.

c. MIAVR has been criticized for the high cost associated with the setting up of a unit of minimally invasive surgery. But these costs are more likely to be compensated by shorter ICU and hospital stays, less blood transfusion requirements and fewer post-operative complications.

d. There is also known morbidity associated with peripheral cannulation. It may be associated with a wound infection, pseudo aneurysm formation, limb ischemia and neurological complications [35].

10. The future

Developments in minimally invasive techniques could potentially lead to totally endoscopic aortic valve replacement (TEAVR) as standard of care for aortic valve replacement [36]. It aims to avoid any sternal fracture or costal spreading by decreasing iatrogenic chest wall trauma. It also aims to maintain advantages of a surgical approach over TAVI. Suture less bio prosthesis technologies are essential to do valve replacement procedures using trocars.

11. Conclusion

MIAVR using RAMT or MS is a safe and effective procedure with excellent post-operative outcomes. Although cross clamp and CPB times may be longer than conventional AVR, use of suture less valve may increase the permeation of MIAVR in the cardiac surgery community. MIAVR with suture less bio prosthesis may be a real alternative to TAVI for the high risk operable patient.

Conflict of interest

The authors have no conflict of interest.

Abbreviations and acronyms

AVR	aortic valve replacement
CPB	cardiopulmonary bypass
MIAVR	minimally invasive aortic valve replacement
MS	mini-sternotomy
RAMT	right anterior mini-thoracotomy
TEAVR	total endoscopic aortic valve replacement
SVC	superior vena cava
TOE	trans oesophageal echocardiography
ABG	arterial blood gas

Author details

Imran Khan[1], Julian A. Smith[1*] and Naresh Trehan[2]

1 Department of Cardiothoracic Surgery, Monash Health and Department of Surgery, School of Clinical Sciences at Monash Health, Monash University, Clayton, Victoria, Australia

2 Medanta Heart Institute, Gurgaon, India

*Address all correspondence to: julian.smith@monash.edu

References

[1] Holzhey D, Mohr FW, Walther T, Mollmann H, Beckmann A, et al. Current results of surgical aortic valve replacement: Insights from the german aortic valve registry. The Annals of Thoracic Surgery. 2016;**101**:658-666

[2] Joshi P, Doshi C, Vinchurkar M, Thosani R, Mahajan SV. Minimally invasive combined aortic and mitral valve replacement. Heart, Lung and Circulation. 2011;**20**(4):231-233

[3] Cosgrove DM 3rd, Sabik JF. Minimally invasive approach for aortic valve operation. The Annals of Thoracic Surgery. 1996;**62**:596-597

[4] Bennetti FJ, Mariana MA, Rizzardi JL, Bennetti I. Minimally invasive aortic valve replacement. The Journal of Thoracic and Cardiovascular Surgery. 1997;**113**:806-807

[5] Gundry SR, Shattuch OH, Razzouk AJ, Del Rio MJ, Sarawu FF. Facile minimally invasive cardiac surgery via ministernotomy. The Annals of Thoracic Surgery. 1998;**65**:1100-1104

[6] Marcovola FJF, Campisi S, Faure M, Sandri F. Totally endoscopic aortic valve replacement (TEAVR). Annals of cardiothoracic surgery. 2015;**4**(2):196-197

[7] Beckmann A, Funkat AK, Lewandowski J, Frie M, Ernst M, et al. German heart surgery report 2016: The annual updated registry of the german society for thoracic and cardiovascular surgery. The Thoracic and Cardiovascular Surgeon. 2017;**65**:505-518

[8] Hamm CW, Mollman H, Holzhey D, Beckmann A, Veit C, Figulla HR, et al. The german aortic valve registry (GARY): In-hospital outcome. European Heart Journal. 2014;**35**:1588-1598

[9] Kaneko T, Vassileva CM, Englum B, Kim S, Yanmie M, Brennan M, et al. Contemporary outcomes of repeat aortic valve replacement: A benchmark for transcatheter valve-in-valve procedures. The Annals of Thoracic Surgery. 2015;**100**:1298-1304

[10] Thourani VH, Borger MA, Holmes D, Maniar H, Pinto F, et al. Transatlantic commentary on transcatheter aortic valve replacement. Journal of Thoracic and Cardiovascular Surgery. 2017;**52**:1-13

[11] Glauber M, Gilmanov D, Farneti PA, Kalluski E, Miceli A, et al. Right anterior minithoracotomy for aortic valve replacement: 10 year experience of a single centre. The Journal of Thoracic and Cardiovascular Surgery. 2015;**150**:548-556

[12] Schmitto JD, Mokashi SA, Cohn LH. Minimally invasive valve surgery. American College of Cardiology. 2010;**56**:455-462

[13] Rosengart K, Feldman T, Borger MA, et al. Percutaneous and minimally invasive valve procedures: A scientific statement from the american heart association council on cardiovascular surgery and anaesthesia, council on clinical cardiology, functional genomics and translational biology, interdisciplinary working group and quality of care and outcomes research interdisciplinary working group. Circulation. 2008;**117**:1750-1767

[14] STS National Database Spring 2003, Executive Summary. Durham, NC: Duke Clinical Research Institute; 2003

[15] Tabata M, Fukui T, Takanashi S. Do minimally invasive approaches improve outcomes of heart valve surgery? Circulation Journal. 2013;77:2232-2239

[16] Khoshbin E, Prayaga S, Kinsella J, Sutherland FW. Mini-sternotomy for aortic valve replacement reduces the

length of stay in cardiac intensive care unit: Met analysis of randomized control trials. BMJ Open. 2011;**1**:e000266

[17] Phan K, Xie A, Di Eusanio M, Yan TD. A meta-analysis of minimally invasive versus conventional sternotomy for aortic valve replacement. The Annals of Thoracic Surgery. 2014;**98**:1499-1511

[18] Burdett CL, Lage IB, Goodwin AT, White RW, Khan KJ, et al. Manubrium—Limited sternotomy decreases blood loss after aortic valve replacement surgery. Interactive Cardiovascular and Thoracic Surgery. 2014;**19**(4):605-610

[19] Borger M, Vladim M, Lenard C, Knosalla C, Markus R, et al. A randomized multicenter trial of minimally invasive rapid deployment versus conventional full sternotomy aortic valve replacement. The Annals of Thoracic Surgery. 2015;**99**:17-25

[20] Brown ML, Mckellar SH, Sundt TM, Schaff HV. Ministernotomy versus conventional sternotomy for aortic valve replacement: A systemic review and meta-analysis. The Journal of Thoracic and Cardiovascular Surgery. 2009;**137**:670.e5-679.e5

[21] Stolinski J, Musial R, Plicner D, Andres J. Respiratory system function after minimally invasive aortic valve replacement surgery. A case control study. Innovations. 2017;**12**(2):127-136

[22] Ghanta RK, Lapar DJ, Kern JA, Kron IL, Speir AM, et al. Minimally invasive aortic valve replacement provides equivalent outcomes at reduced cost compared with conventional aortic valve replacement: A real-world multi-institutional analysis. The Journal of Thoracic and Cardiovascular Surgery. 2015;**149**(4):1060-1065

[23] Lamellas. Minimally invasive aortic valve replacement: The "Miami Method". Annals of cardiothoracic surgery. 2015;**4**(1):71-77

[24] Von Segesser LK, Westaby S, Pomar J, Loisance D, Groscurta P, et al. Less invasive aortic valve surgery: Rational & technique. European Journal of Cardio-Thoracic Surgery. 1999;**15**:781-785

[25] Shaalan AM, Kasbi I, Elwakeel EE, Elkamali YA. Outcome of surgical repair of pectus excavatum in adults. Journal of Cardiothoracic Surgery. 2017;**12**:72

[26] Toledano B, Bisbal P, Camara ML, Labata C, Berastequi E, et al. Incidence and predictors of new onset atrioventricular block requiring pacemaker implantation after sutureless aortic valve replacement. Interactive Cardiovascular and Thoracic Surgery. 2016;**23**:861-868

[27] Murtuza B, Pepper JL, Stanbridge RD, et al. Minimal access aortic valve replacement: Is it worth it? The Annals of Thoracic Surgery. 2008;**85**:1121-1131

[28] Glauber E, Micelli A, Bevilacqua S, et al. Minimally invasive aortic valve replacement via right anterior minithoracotomy: Early outcomes and midterm follow up. The Journal of Thoracic and Cardiovascular Surgery. 2011;**142**:1577-1579

[29] Micelli A, Murzi M, Gilmanov D, Fuga R, Ferrarini M, et al. Minimally invasive aortic valve replacement using right minithoracotomy is associated with better outcomes than ministernotomy. The Journal of Thoracic and Cardiovascular Surgery. 2014;**148**:133-137

[30] Tabata M, Umakanthan R, Khalpey Z, et al. Coversion to full sternotomy during minimal access cardiac surgery: Reasons and results during a 9.5 year experience. The Journal of Thoracic and Cardiovascular Surgery. 2007;**134**:165-169

[31] Folliguet TA, Laborde F, Zannis K, et al. Sutureless Perceval aortic valve replacement: Results of two European

centres. The Annals of Thoracic Surgery. 2012;**93**:1483-1488

[32] Kocher AA, Laufer G, Haverich A, et al. One year outcomes of the surgical treatment of aortic stenosis with a next generation surgical aortic valve (TRITON) trial: A prospective multicenter study of rapid—Deployment aortic valve replacement with the EDWARDS INTUITY valve system. The Journal of Thoracic and Cardiovascular Surgery. 2013;**145**:110-115; discussion 115-6

[33] Micelli A, Santarpino G, Pfeiffer S, et al. Minimally invasive aortic valve replacement with Perceval S sutureless valve: Early outcomes and one year survival from two European centres. The Journal of Thoracic and Cardiovascular Surgery. 2014;**148**:2838-2843

[34] Santarpino G, Pfeiffer S, Jessi J, et al. Sutureless replacement versus transcatheter valve implantation in aortic valve stenosis: A propensity matched analysis of 2 strategies in high risk patients. The Journal of Thoracic and Cardiovascular Surgery. 2014;**147**:561-567

[35] Murzi M, Cerillo AG, Miceli A, et al. Antegrade and retrograde arterial perfusion strategy in minimally invasive mitral-valve surgery: A propensity score analysis on 1280 patients. European Journal of Cardio-Thoracic Surgery. 2013;**43**:e167-e172

[36] Vola M, Fuzelier JF, Chavent B, et al. First human totally endoscopic aortic valve replacement: An early report. The Journal of Thoracic and Cardiovascular Surgery. 2014;**147**:1091-1093

Chapter 6

Minimally Invasive Approach in Surgery for Congenital Heart Disease

Massimo A. Padalino, Demetrio G. Pittarello, Vladimiro L. Vida and Giovanni Stellin

Abstract

Surgery for congenital heart disease (CHD) has changed considerably during the last decade. Improved surgical results in patients with simple CHD and new interventional cardiology procedures have stimulated the surgeon to adopt minimally invasive techniques to reduce the patient's surgical insult and obtain good functional and cosmetic results. As a consequence, new surgical techniques and specialized equipment for minimally invasive cardiac surgery (MICS) procedures have been developed and refined in recent years. The improving surgical outcomes in patients with CHD, the significant advances in surgical instrumentation and perfusion technology, and the broad utilization of new catheter-based interventional procedures to repair simple CHD have triggered surgeons' interest to adopt and innovate minimally invasive approaches for CHD repair, so as to reduce patient's surgical trauma and improve functional and cosmetic results while maintaining a high standard of clinical outcomes and possibly shortening hospitalization times. This article reports on our updated full experience and institutional protocols with MICS in children and adults with CHD.

Keywords: congenital heart defects, minimally invasive, surgery, long-term outcomes, cost-effective

1. Introduction

Ever since the first intracardiac repair of an atrial septal defect (ASD) by Lewis and Varco in 1954 [1], congenital heart surgery has continued to evolve, to become a widely available treatment modality with excellent results. Simple defects like an ASD can now be repaired with almost no mortality and morbidity. In the meantime, interventional cardiology has developed significantly effective transcatheter procedures to perform therapeutic closure of simple defects as well as relieving valvar and vascular obstructions. These catheter-based repairs as an alternative to the surgical gold standard have become popular thanks to its minimally invasive appeal and excellent cosmetic outcome. However, sometimes results may be suboptimal [2, 3], and they may also have severe postoperative complications leading to death [4]. However, these procedures are equally well accepted because they are claimed to be "noninvasive. "Despite the current advancement of surgical and catheter-based techniques having been pursued for the patient's benefit, as physicians and surgeon,

IntechOpen

we have to remember that our goal is to accomplish the optimal repair that ensures a healthy survival, a safe technique, and the best quality of life, either physical or psychological.

There are several surgical approaches that have been proposed as an alternative to the standard sternotomy [5] which have been introduced to reduce the invasiveness of surgery while ensuring the perfect repair. In addition, since a sternal scar, however small, continues to be at a disadvantage because of it attracting a stigma of being a cardiac patient or because of sociocultural issues, other alternatives must be explored. These have included a small incision with a full sternotomy [6], a partial sternotomy or mini-sternotomy [7, 8], a right axillary [9] or anterolateral [10, 11], as well as a posterior thoracotomy [12–14]. However, as more experience was gained, the complete anterolateral thoracotomy (in spite of being once considered superior to a sternotomy) has been less utilized because of reports of thoracic cage deformity (caused by rib deformation and atrophy of severed pectoral muscles) and asymmetric development of breasts when used prepubescently [15]. Utilization of a mini-anterolateral thoracotomy and an appropriate location of the incision away from the nipple area have been reported by our group to avoid these complications in the long term [16, 17].

Thus, the improving surgical outcomes in patients with CHD, the significant advances in surgical instrumentation and perfusion technology, and the broad utilization of new catheter-based interventional procedures to repair simple CHD have triggered surgeons' interest to adopt and innovate minimally invasive approaches for CHD repair, so as to reduce the patient's surgical trauma and improve functional and cosmetic results while maintaining a high standard of clinical outcomes and possibly shortening hospitalization times.

We present our current experience with MICS in patients with CHD, according to our institutional policy.

2. The Padova minimally invasive congenital cardiac surgery protocol

Since the early 1990s, we have continuously adopted a minimally invasive approach to the surgical closure of simple CHD which has evolved through the years to a systematic protocol of MICS for all patients with simple and moderately severe CHD, which includes:

- Routine perioperative transesophageal 2D-echo monitoring (TEE); in small infants weighing less than 4 kg, we have used epicardial 2D echocardiography.
- Postoperative pain control.
- "FastTrack" management (extubation within 3 hours of mechanical ventilation).
- Early discharge from the intensive care unit (ICU).
- Early discharge home (within 4–5 days from the operation) [16].

The surgical approach has always been chosen according to the patient's age, gender, and specific patient's request, balancing safety and effectiveness of the operation and patient's satisfaction after the operation (according to the "gender-differentiated minimally invasive surgery" protocol [7]). For example, a right anterior mini-thoracotomy (RAMT) is less visible in adult females when the incision is within the submammary sulcus. An axillary lateral mini-thoracotomy (RALMT) is currently offered to both male and females whose weight is higher than 10 kg, for repair of simple CHD such as ASD, partial anomalous pulmonary venous drainage (PAPVD), discrete subaortic stenosis (SAS), membranous ventricular septal defect (VSD), and partial atrioventricular septal defects (p-AVSD). On the contrary, some kind of a mini-sternotomy (MS), meant as limited to the body of the sternum, is offered mostly to infants and children, weighing less than 10 kg, in order to repair lesions other than ASD, such as large VSD with significant left to right shunt in 3–6-month-old infants. In fact, according to our experience, this approach with the help of an appropriate retractor (Bookwalker retractor, Codman Surgical instruments, GS Medical Ltd., Dublin) can guarantee an excellent exposure of the great vessels when other maneuvers are required (i.e., aortic cross-clamping, pulmonary valvotomy, closure of patent ductus arteriosus (PDA)). In addition to these approaches, a right posterior mini-thoracotomy (RPMT) has occasionally been offered as a surgical option in older children and young females, to approach the aortic valve, SAS repair, and VSD closure. Also, from June 2006, as a refinement of our minimally invasive protocol, we have routinely employed peripheral cannulation (usually through right groin vessels) for the cardiopulmonary bypass in patients with simple CHD and a bodyweight superior to 15 kg.

Last, as part of our minimally invasive armamentarium, a video-assisted thoracoscopic surgery (VATS) has also been widely utilized since 1994, for the correction of simple CHD as PDA and vascular rings. However, after the introduction of percutaneous closure of restrictive PDA, we have drastically reduced this practice.

2.1 Transesophageal echocardiography

Routine TEE imaging is helpful in the surgical repair of CHD in children. Performance of TEE in these patients submitted to MICS represents a great contributor to the overall excellence in outcome for CHD. The TEE that has been used intraoperatively since the 1980s [17, 18] is a mainstay of monitoring during simple and complex pediatric cardiovascular surgery [19, 20], especially in MICS, since it provides dynamic control and intraoperative anatomical information but also:

- Allows the surgeon to review the anatomical findings preoperatively.
- Can diagnose myocardial performance.
- Provides an evaluation of postsurgical results and can show residual shunts or other surgical problems that can be addressed during the same operative time (avoiding repeat surgery and its associated costs [21, 22]).
- Allows evaluation of effective de-airing after MICS procedure, enhancing patient's safety in regard to air embolism-related problems.

It has been especially valuable in the operating room where it is used preoperatively to confirm or modify anatomical diagnoses which have been established by TTE and angiography and also identifies possible additional pathologic conditions to delineate anatomy and structural details that may have remained ill-defined by transthoracic imaging [23–25]. The technological advancements, particularly the use of small probe sizes, have significantly improved patient safety and success of cardiac surgery in infants and children [26–33].

The probe is usually inserted by the anesthesiologist, after induction of general anesthesia, and it is used for all the time of operation with a Philips Sonos IE33 echocardiography machines (Philips, Andover, MA) equipped with pulsed, continuous wave, color Doppler, and 3D capabilities. In patients >20 kg, we have been using an adult probe (xMatrix probe: X7-2t; 3D matrix array probe; 2–7 MHz; Philips, Andover, MA) with 2500 elements per transducer and, on the contrary, in pediatric patients (whose weight is between 4.0 and 20.0 kg), a pediatric probe (Mini Multi probe: S7-3t; 3–7 MHz; Philips, Andover, MA) with 64 elements per transducer and dimensions of 10.7 mm (tip width) and 8.0 mm (tip height).

These clinical benefits, a growing number of highly skilled operators, and improvements in technology have led to the rapid adoption of TEE monitoring in pediatric cardiac surgery with remarkable advances in the management of patients with congenital heart disease in this particular setting.

2.2 Anesthesia care

In recent years, "FastTrack" management (FTM), in the perioperative care of patients with CHD, with early tracheal extubation after cardiac surgery, has become increasingly popular [34–37] especially in MICS, with the delivery of cost-efficient care considered as an additional variable when measuring and comparing surgical outcomes [37, 38].

Potential advantages were previously described [38]:

1. Reduced incidence of airway irritation and ventilator-associated complications (i.e., accidental extubation, laryngotracheal trauma, pulmonary hypertensive crisis during endotracheal tube suctioning, mucous plugging of endotracheal tubes, barotraumas secondary to positive airway pressure ventilation, and ventilator-associated pulmonary infections and atelectasis)

2. Reduced parental stress

3. Reduced requirements of sedation and potential associated hemodynamic compromise

4. More rapid patient mobilization

5. Earlier ICU discharge

6. Decreased length of hospital stay

7. Reduced costs (ventilator-associated and length of ICU/hospital stay)

In this context, anesthesia should not be managed by a strict protocol. A general institutional approach for children who are candidates to FastTrack extubation consisted of induction of anesthesia with thiopental 5 mg/kg, fentanyl 3 mcg/kg, and rocuronium 0.9 mg/kg. During surgery and cardiopulmonary bypass (CPB), anesthesia is maintained with remifentanil 0.5–1 mcg/kg/min and propofol 3–5 mg/kg. Muscle relaxants are given again before CPB at 0.15 mg/kg. The patient is monitored as routine (ECG, pulse oximetry, invasive arterial pressure, central venous pressure, diuresis, temperature, and somatic and cerebral near-infrared spectroscopy (NIRS)). Shortly before the end of the surgery, remifentanil is discontinued, and intravenous morphine (0.1–0.2 mg/kg) or fentanyl (1–2 mcg/kg) is administered. When surgery is over, according to FTM protocol, the neuromuscular block is reversed by the intravenous administration of atropine, 0.01 mg/kg, and neostigmine, 0.05 mg/kg. Immediate post-extubation analgesia or sedation in children includes a single administration of rectal paracetamol (40–50 mg/kg), a bolus of morphine 0.05 mg/kg iv or fentanyl 0.5–1 mcg/kg iv, and/or midazolam 0.05–1 mg/kg iv, with repeated boluses as needed.

For the first 24 postoperative hours, morphine is given by continuous iv in most patients. Pain scores and vital signs are recorded by the bedside nurse, on an hourly basis throughout the day, or, when appropriate, by the parents or even by the child, if it is old enough to report his/her pain scores on a 0–10 pain scale. Supplemental analgesia is administrated if required, according to the recorded pain scores.

Despite this program, extubation in the OR after pediatric cardiac surgery is to be meditated. In order to migrate to a routine practice of early extubation, it is necessary that surgeons, anesthesiologists, intensivists, perfusionists, and nurses have the same mindset and cooperate to achieve this goal and the final decision. Extubation, either in the operating room or in the ICU, is usually decided based on clinical evaluation and also considering some operative parameters such as bypass and aortic cross-clamp times, the complexity of surgery, requirement of high dosage inotropic support, hemodynamic stability, and occurrence of persistent bleeding. Operating room extubation is usually not performed if there are signs of airway compromise, hemodynamic instability requiring bolus delivery of vasopressors, cardiac rhythm instability, excessive bleeding, or core temperature < 35°C.

In patients submitted to VATS, postoperative pain is significant, especially early after surgery [39, 40], and higher than sternotomy. For these reasons, there has been an increased interest in the use of paravertebral block (PVB). The intercostal nerves are relatively devoid of covering fascia as they traverse the paravertebral space, making it an ideal location for local anesthetic blockade [41]. The PVB technique includes the use of ultrasound [42] with a linear probe at high frequency in pediatric patient with weight > 15 kg, alternatively, which can be performed by a single injection at the level of paravertebral space intraoperatively under direct vision by the surgeon [43] or anesthesiologists prior to chest closure [44]. The single-shot multilevel PVB with ropivacaine 0.5% has a place in these procedures (max 0.4 ml/kg at the fifth intercostal space), with analgesic benefits seen in the first few hours, and can reduce long-term adverse pain outcomes.

In this kind of patients, a change in the attitude of surgeons, anesthesiologists, perfusionists, and nurses, combined with appropriate anesthetic and surgical techniques, permitted better results and outcomes.

2.3 Cardiopulmonary bypass and operative strategies

According to our minimally invasive surgical protocol [45], a direct aortic and bicaval cannulation is usually employed in patients with a body weight of less than 10 kg. Since 2006, in larger patients, we have routinely used a peripheral arterial and venous cannulation [46–48] for establishing the cardiopulmonary bypass (CPB). This is achieved by percutaneous cannulation of the superior vena cava (SVC) followed by surgical isolation and cannulation of the femoral vessels (**Figure 1**).

The SVC peripheral cannulation is usually performed by a trained anesthesiologist with experience with patients with CHD, using 2D transesophageal echo (TEE) guidance (**Figure 2**), after 100 U/kg of heparin has been systemically administered [46]. The internal jugular vein is punctured and dilated, and then an SVC (Medtronic Biomedicus 96,570 Next Gen, MN, USA) is inserted and positioned under TEE monitoring, about 1 cm above the SVC-right atrial junction. Currently, we reserve this approach to DVAPP, in which the presence of pulmonary veins in the SVC may complicate the traditional SVC cannulation through a small incision. In all other cases, as experience has increased, we have recently moved to a direct SVC cannulation with a right angle metal tipped venous cannula (Medtronic DLP single

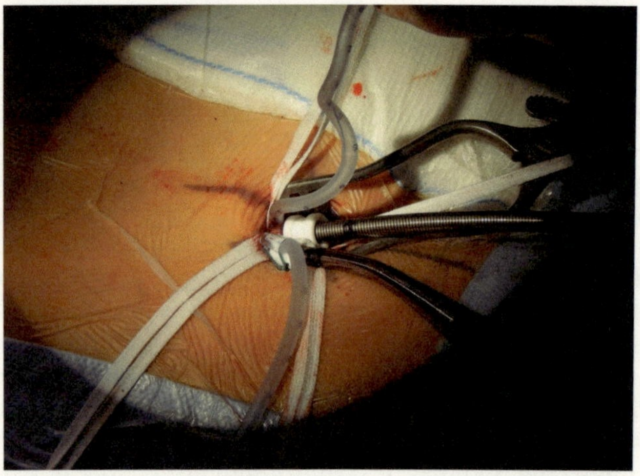

Figure 1.
Exposure of the femoral artery and vein is obtained by means of a transversal skin incision (2 cm in length) along with the groin folder (bikini incision).

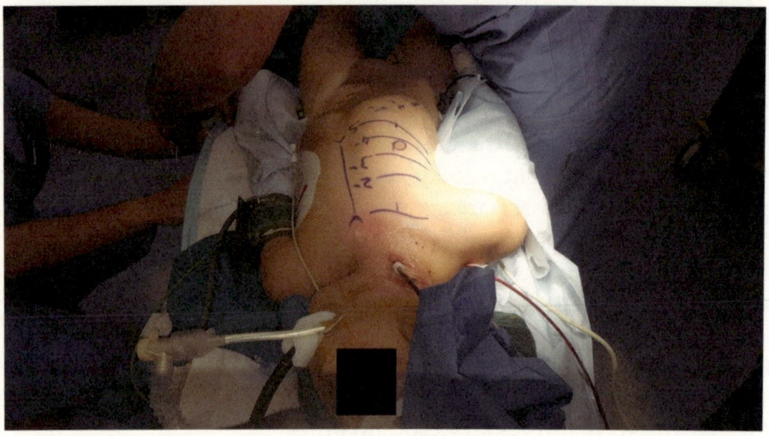

Figure 2.
Percutaneous cannulation of the internal jugular vein utilizing a venous cannula (bio-Medicus Medtronic, USA), inserted using standard echo-guided modified Seldinger technique.

stage venous) through a usual 5.0 Prolene purse string on the right atrium or in the SVC when approach is through an ALT, where SVC is very well exposed (**Figure 3**).

A 2 cm incision is employed at the inguinal fold (**Figure 1**) for exposing the femoral artery and vein. After full systemic heparinization has been achieved (with activated clotting time (ACT) > 400 s), direct arterial cannulation is usually accomplished with a femoral arterial cannula with introducer (Medtronic Biomedicus 96,570 NextGen MN, USA). Venous cannulation (Medtronic Biomedicus 96,670 NextGen MN, USA femoral venous cannula) is then performed using the Seldinger technique under TEE guidance that can clearly show the guide in the right atrium.

In children weighing less than 15 kg, the femoral artery may be too small for safe cannulation; for this reason, we prefer central cannulation in the ascending aorta, utilizing a FEM FLEX arterial cannula, fixed with double 4.0 Ticron purse string. This mixed cannulation approach has allowed us to extend MICS to children as small as 10 kg.

When femoral arterial cannulation is performed, we routinously monitor both lower extremities by NIRS, with sensors positioned on the anterior side of the thigh,

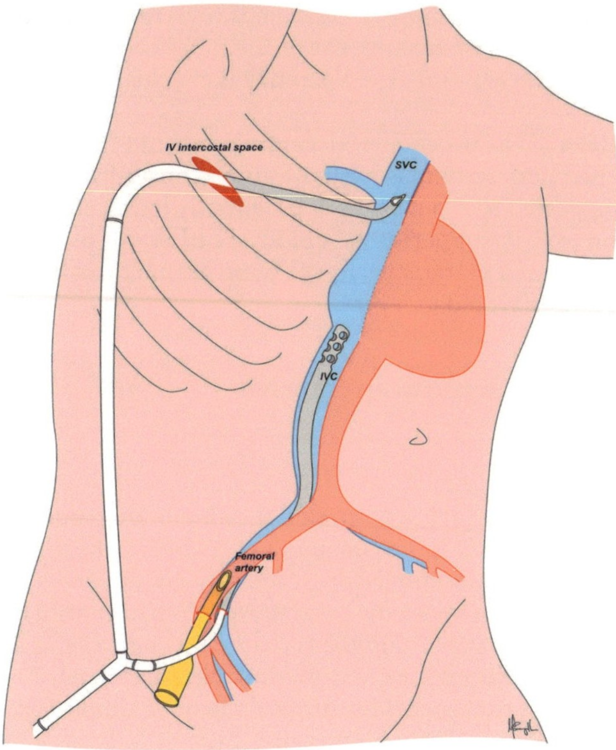

Figure 3.
Diagram showing direct superior vena cava cannulation through the RALMT, with a right angle metal tipped venous cannula.

so as to check for any oxygen saturation variations in the cannulated leg during the extracorporeal perfusion [48].

Assisted venous drainage (with a maximum vacuum of 50 mmHg) is adopted to minimize the size of tubing and venous cannulas (that are usually one to two under the estimated size for a patient's body surface area [BSA]). Once the cardiopulmonary bypass is started, mild hypothermia (rectal temperature of 34–35°C) is reached [45].

At full flow, once the venae cavae are snared, ventricular fibrillation is induced by an epicardial electrode and cable connected to a fibrillator (Fi 20 M, Stockert, Livanova Group, Munich, Germany) in all patients requiring a RAMT. On the contrary, when a MS or RPMT is used, a conventional aortic cross-clamping with cold hematic cardioplegia may be employed as an alternative.

At the end of the intracardiac repair, an accurate de-airing of the left cardiac sections is performed under transesophageal 2D-echocardiographic monitoring, on Trendelenburg position. The de-airing is obtained by filling the left cardiac chambers with saline solution before declamping or defibrillating. Sustained blow ventilation is always performed by the anesthesiologist to clear the left atrial chamber from residual air bubbles. During induced ventricular fibrillation time, it is essential to avoid blood suction inside the left cardiac sections.

After surgical repair is completed and the intracardiac de-airing is completed, the induced fibrillation is discontinued. An intravenous lidocaine bolus of 1 mg/kg is given, and the heart is promptly defibrillated by external direct current shock (3–5 J/kg) when sinus rhythm is not naturally restored. In patients requiring aortic cross-clamping, a further de-bubbling is achieved through the cardioplegia needle by continuous suction, before and after clamp removal.

At the end of CPB, systemic heparinization is reverted, and the femoral cannulas are then removed. After chest closure, the SVC cannula is removed by the anesthesiologist. As a routine, the femoral vessel patency is checked by 2D-echo and Doppler, before discharge.

After completion of the procedure, decannulation and hemostasis are performed. The opened pericardium is partially approximated with interrupted stitches; this is suggested to avoid rare but potentially lethal complications such as cardiac herniation [49]. A subperiosteal epidural catheter is placed in the posterior intercostal groove created extrapleurally for bupivacaine infusion. A thorax drain is inserted and the thorax closed in layers.

3. Minimally invasive surgical approaches

3.1 Mini-sternotomy

As previously described [45], a 4-cm skin incision in the midline of the chest, with its superior margin at or approximately 1–2 cm below the nipple level, is employed (**Figure 4**). The sternum is longitudinally divided in its lower third, up to its body and retracted to expose the great vessels. When central cannulation is employed, the inferior vena cava cannula is passed through a separate 5-mm skin incision (which is later utilized for the chest drainage insertion).

The MS approach is usually used for surgical repair of simple CHD lesions as ASD, VSD, PAPVD, and p-AVSD in infants and children. Whenever the child is older than 5 years, the sternal bone is more rigid, and the simple MS may not allow a safe exposure of ascending aorta. For this reason, we usually utilize a T-incision (**Figure 5**) which consists in an extension of the midline sternal incision about 5–10 mm laterally (right and left) at the level of the third intercostal space, without reaching the external border of the sternal body and the mammary artery. This incision can be safely performed with an oscillatory saw. The application of a reverse T mini-sternotomy has also been applied to young adults for aortic valve repair or replacement, with or without associated ascending aorta vascular graft replacement. The right pleura is routinely opened, and the pericardium is incised laterally down to 1 cm from the right phrenic nerve to create a sort of pericardial window, to avoid possible cardiac tamponade in case of severe postoperative pericardial effusion.

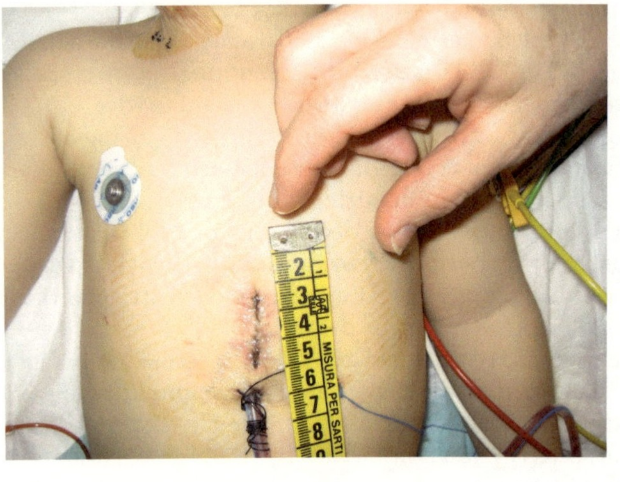

Figure 4.
Mini-sternotomy approach: The cutaneous incision (3–5 cm long) is done below the line between the two nipples.

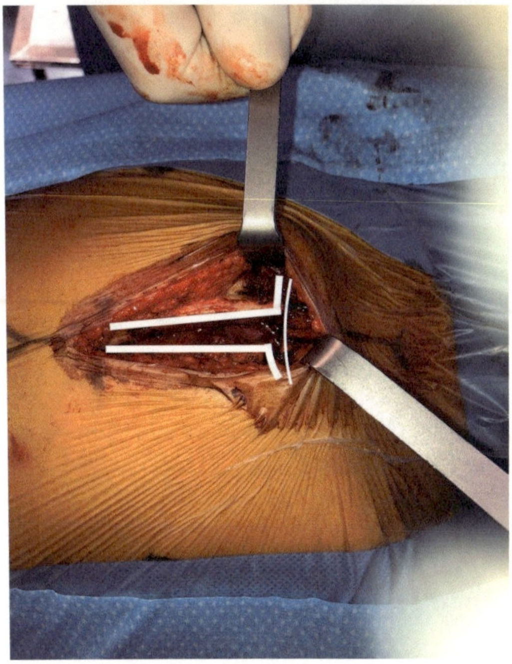

Figure 5.
T-sternal incision mini-sternotomy (T-MT) is useful in older children to expose the great vessels adequately.

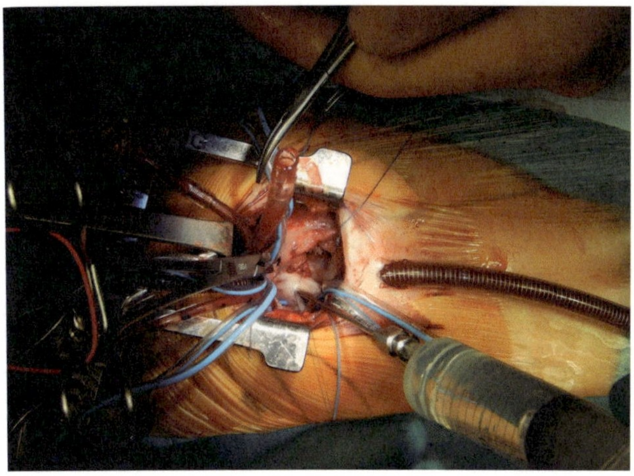

Figure 6.
Right anterior mini-thoracotomy approach.

3.2 Right anterior mini-thoracotomy

We use this technique mainly in female patients (some children but mostly teenagers and adults) for ostium secundum type ASD closure, as an alternative to an MS. In RAMT, a 4-cm semilunar incision in the sulcus of the right breast is entering the chest in the fourth intercostal space (**Figure 6**). In the prepuberty age, the incision is kept very low under the right nipple (at about 5–8 cm away from the nipple area [7, 16]), particularly in female patients, to avoid any possible future interference with breast development [45]. Subcutaneous fat and mammary gland are gently dissected from the fascia up to the fourth intercostal space, where the chest cavity is entered. The incision of the intercostal space is approximately 1 cm longer than the skin incision at each side. A video-assisted optical technology using a 5 mm 0° optical scope, which is inserted through a separate 5 mm incision, in the fourth intercostal space, may be helpful to implement the surgical vision [45], but with increased experience we have realized that this aid is rarely necessary for infants and children. In patients >15 kg who undergo peripheral cannulation, the SVC is usually occluded with a cross-clamp that is inserted through a separate lateral 5-mm incision that is later utilized for inserting chest drainage.

3.3 Right posterior mini-thoracotomy

In our hands, this approach has been ideal for treating discrete SAS, PAPVD, and sinus venosus ASD. This technique was introduced for simple CHD since 2001. After the original description by Metras and Kreitmann in 1999 [14] for repairing simple CHD, we have modified it from a classic wide right posterior thoracotomy to a mini-thoracotomy, the RPMT (**Figure 7**). Currently, a 4-cm subscapular incision is employed for entering the chest in the fourth intercostal space [45]. This technique has been mainly used in female patients (under specific patient's request). Through this surgical approach, the aorta can be easily visualized and cross-clamped, and aortic valve area can be exposed.

3.4 Right axillary lateral mini-thoracotomy

The right axillary lateral mini-thoracotomy is currently out the approach of choice since it can be safely and efficiently employed for repair of various types of moderately severe CHD, similar to standard surgical procedures, either in adults or in children as small as 10 kg. A right axillary incision provides the best direct plane of vision to the atrial septum, AV valves, and the membranous ventricular septum (**Figure 8**). On the contrary, we do not suggest this approach for conal septal defects or pulmonary valve procedures, since the right ventricular outflow tract is not accessible to expose, and there is the potential risk of a suboptimal repair and postoperative residual defects or complications. Also, the axillary area is one of the least muscularly covered parts of the thoracic cage, allowing for less invasive transthoracic access to the heart. Last, the subaxillary location of the scar, being far away from the breast and being naturally covered by a resting arm, provides an excellent cosmetic result, either in female or in male patients. At the beginning of our experience, we primarily employed this approach to close ostium secundum type ASD. As

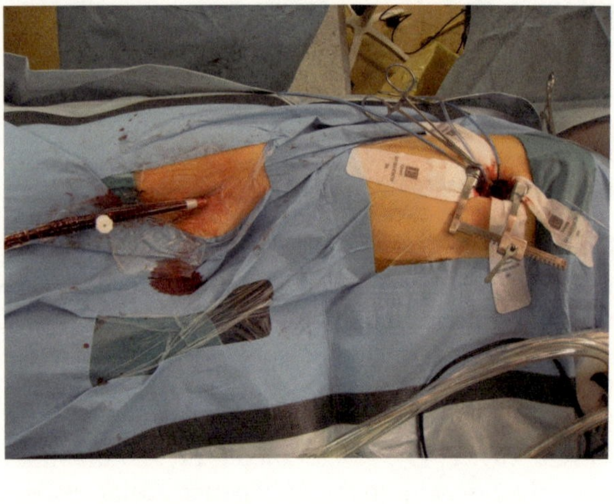

Figure 7.
Right axillary lateral mini-thoracotomy approach.

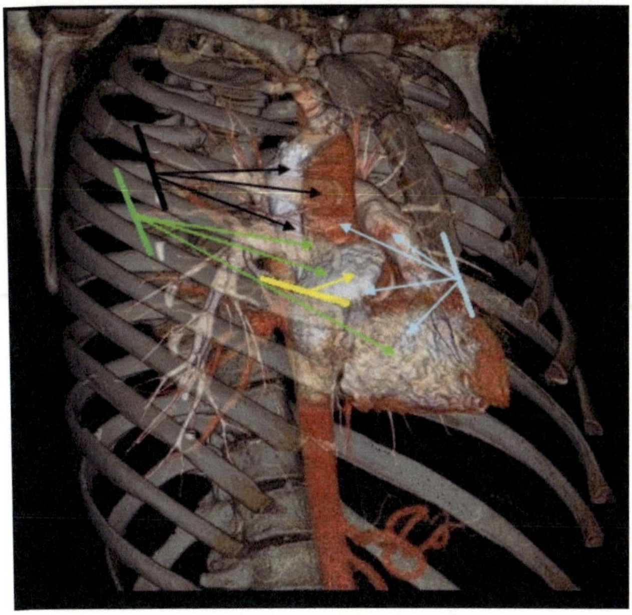

Figure 8.
Minimal invasive approaches and cardiac structure exposure. Angio-CT scan 3D reconstruction in a control patient (right oblique anterior view) showing different minimally invasive surgical chest approaches and their relationship with the cardiac structures and their related capability of exposing them adequately: (A) mini-sternotomy (light blue) shows atrial and ventricular septa and the great vessels. (B) Right anterior mini-thoracotomy (yellow) shows atrial septum; (C) right axillary lateral mini-thoracotomy to perform various procedures on the superior vena cava and aorta through III intercostal space (black) and on the atrial or membranous ventricular septa through the IV intercostal space (green).

we gained experience and confidence about exposure of various parts of the heart, application of this approach has been extended to the correction of other CHD, such as PAPVC of right-sided pulmonary veins (including performance of the Warden procedure—SVC reinsertion onto the RA appendage), the scimitar vein syndrome (off pump relocation of the anomalous vein to the left atrium), partial AVSD, SAS, and restrictive peri-membranous/subaortic VSD.

The patient is placed in a left lateral decubitus, with slightly backward reclining position. The lower torso and pelvic region are placed in a 45-degree position to allow access to the inguinal region (**Figure 9**). Marked anterior and median axillary lines and the appropriate intercostal space are used as guiding parameters for the proper axillary incision. In fact, a third intercostal space may be better for DVAPP repair, since it allows a perfect exposure of the entire SVC area to the innominate vein, while a fourth or fifth intercostal space is better indicated for ASD or VSD or mitral valve exposure. An oblique incision is performed in the right axilla from the median to the anterior line, not extending the latter one. The skin is undermined to be able to slide to the desired operative field. The latissimus dorsi is mobilized free of its fascial attachments, and the digitations of serratus anterior overlying the intercostal space are identified and split. The thoracothomy is performed with a subperiosteal entry through the superior margin of the rib. The pericardium is opened 2 cm anterior to the phrenic nerve. Placing stay sutures along both the margins of the pericardium should be placed so as to expose the field as much as possible. Sometimes, the institution of CPB through inguinal cannulation and deflation of the lungs are necessary to achieve adequate exposure of the heart. In patients older than 15 years or weighing more than 25 kg, a selective bronchial intubation is feasible and highly recommended so as to deflate the right lung and keep the left lung inflated during the procedure (whose inflated volume can push

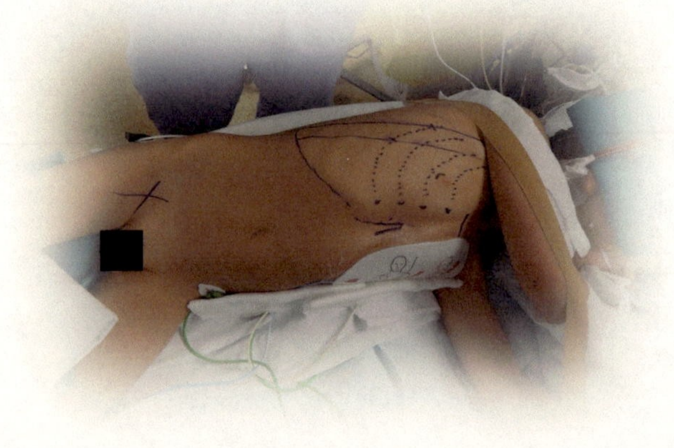

Figure 9.
Operative position of the patient undergoing a RALMT; the patient is rotated in left lateral decubitus, and the proposed incision lines are shown.

up the heart and allow for a better exposure of the surgical field). This is especially true in adults with big chest or overweight patients.

3.5 Left posterior extrapleural mini-thoracotomy (LPEMT)

As we have previously reported [45], a left posterior extrapleural mini-thoracotomy may be used for PDA closure [50] as an alternative to VATS closure, according to surgeon's preferences and especially in children with a body weight greater than 3 kg. On a right lateral decubitus position and through a limited left subscapular skin incision (usually 2–3 cm) and total muscle-sparing technique, the superficial thoracic fascia muscularis is incised [50]. The parietal pleura is carefully detached from the thoracic wall with blunt dissection. A triple ligation closes the PDA. The left lung then is re-expanded for preventing air entrapment within the extrapleural space, and the chest is usually closed without the use of chest drainage. This is a straightforward technique that is preferred in patients with a bodyweight of less than 20 kg carrying low postoperative complications when compared with the transpleural approach [50]. This LPEMT procedure with no need for intensive care and hospitalization of only 24 hours has been reported to be cost-effective [50] when compared to traditional transpleural approach, which requires a more extended hospitalization, or to percutaneous procedures, in which the costs of a single or multiple coils, or an Amplatzer device, make costs increase stellarly. In conclusion, the minimally invasive skin and muscle splitting LPEMT technique is a safe and effective procedure, more cosmetic and significantly less expensive than other standard procedures (surgical or percutaneous, respectively).

3.6 Video-assisted thoracoscopy

Video-assisted thoracoscopy has been widely utilized in over 200 patients for PDA closure, before the broad application of percutaneous PDA occlusion. Nowadays, its application is drastically reduced but may be an alternative for infants and children less than 10 kg (or under specific patient's request) [51] and for relieving respiratory/digestive compression caused by vascular rings. Technically, we have described previously this procedure [45]: the patient is put on the right

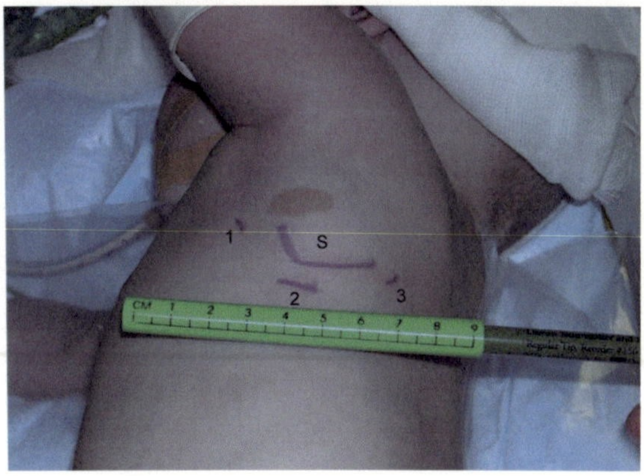

Figure 10.
Patent ductus arteriosus VATS closure. On right decubitus, three mini-incisions are done along with the fourth intercostal space: Two 5-mm long incisions (1 and 3) for the introduction of the surgical instruments in the chest and one 10-mm incision below the tip of the scapula, for the optical camera probe.

lateral decubitus position; three incisions are made around the left scapula (2 of 5 mm and 1 of 10 mm, **Figure 10**). After lung retraction and dissection of the surrounding anatomical structures, a single titanium clip 10 mm long is squeezed tight on the aortic junction of the duct. The complete closure of the duct is routinely assessed in the operating room through cross-sectional and color Doppler echocardiographic imaging, which can be performed with transesophageal or transthoracic echocardiography. In the case of residual shunting, a second clip may be applied. Patients are usually extubated in the operating room and discharged the following day. However, VATS equipment is not everywhere available because of cost considerations.

4. Our 22 years of surgical experience

From 1996 to 2018, we have treated with MICS techniques 976 patients affected by CHD (M/F 387/589). Overall, the median age at repair was 5 years (interquartile range 1.7–11 years). The most common CHD was ASD secundum type in 557 patients (57%), while the remaining were affected by other anomalies (VSD, p-AVSD, PAPVD, SAS). In particular, a large VSD patch closure was performed by MS in 145 infants <1 year of age (14.8%). Minimally invasive access was a midline MS in 452 patients (median age 2, IQR 0.5–5 years), RAMT in 356 (median age 9, IQR 4–20 years), and a RALMT in 168 (median age 9, IQR 6–14 years).

All patients required CPB, and peripheral cannulation was used in 191 patients (19.5%); it is of note that almost all patients undergoing RALMT underwent peripheral cannulation (96%). Induced ventricular fibrillation was used in 598 patients (61.3%), while aortic cross-clamping was employed in the remaining, with a median cross-clamping time of 16 min (IQR 9–25).

There were no early and late deaths at operation. Minor postoperative complications occurred in 110 patients (11.2%), being 39 (35.6%) post-pericardiotomy syndrome. Median intensive care unit stay was 1 day (IQR 1–2), and all patients were discharged home after a median stay of 5 days (IQR 4–6). All clinical preoperative, operative, and postoperative data divided by minimally invasive approach are described in detail in **Table 1**.

Variable (*Patients*)	MS (452)	RAMT (356)	RALMT (168)	p-value
Male*	245 (56)	52 (15)	90 (54)	<0.0001
ASD II*	138 (31)	337 (95)	82 (49)	<0.0001
VSD < 1 aa*	145 (32)	-	-	<0.0001
Other CHD*	169 (37)	19 (5.3)	86 (51)	<0.0001
Age at operation (years)**	2 (0.5-5)	9 (4-20)	9 (6-14)	<0.0001
Age > 18 aa at operation*	6 (1.3)	94 (26)	34 (20)	<0.0001
Weight at operation (kg)**	11 (6-18)	27 (17-52)	30 (19-52)	<0.0001
Peripheral cannulation*	17 (3.8)	103 (29)	161 (96)	<0.0001
CPB time (min)**	70 (43-96)	35 (27-50)	47 (32-71)	<0.0001
ACC*	292 (65)	12 (3.4)	77 (46)	<0.0001
ACC time (min)**	48 (36-60)	37 (32-51)	40 (34-55)	<0.0001
IFV*	161 (36)	344 (97)	93 (55)	<0.0001
IFV time (min)**	14 (9-21)	16 (11-25)	17 (13-25)	<0.0001
ICU stay (days)**	2 (1-2)	1 (1-1)	1 (1-1)	<0.0001
ICU stay > 2 days*	66 (15)	2 (0.6)	2 (1.2)	<0.0001
Total Hospital stay (days)**	5 (4-7)	5 (5-6)	4 (3-5)	<0.0001
Postoperative complications*	71 (16)	18 (5)	21 (13)	<0.0001
Post-pericardiotomy syndrome*	27 (6)	10 (2.8)	2 (1.2)	0.009
Blood transfusion*	208 (46)	37 (10)	3 (1.8)	<0.0001

*number of patients and percentage (%); **median and interquartile range (IQR).

ACC, aortic Cross Clamping; ASD II, atrial septal defect secundum type; CHD, congenital heart disease; CPB, cardio-pulmonary bypass; ICU, intensive care unit; IVF, induced ventricular fibrillation; MS: mini-sternotomy; RALMT, right axillary mini-thoracotomy; RAMT: right anterior mini-thoracotomy; VSD, ventricular septal defect.

Table 1.
Clinical preoperative, operative and postoperative data by minimally invasive approach (n = 976) since 1996.

5. Discussion

Recent technological advances have enabled treatment for a wide range of CHD, with excellent early and late results. As a consequence, both children and adults with CHD can now expect better outcomes. In the last decade, however, surgical techniques have also centered around the reduction of trauma and postoperative recovery time and even improvement of cosmetic results. A standard median sternotomy has been the conventional approach for correction of congenital cardiac defects for many years, but it often yields to unsatisfactory esthetic results [6, 7, 52]. Unsightly midline scars arouse displeasure and psychological distress, especially in young female patients. Minimally invasive cardiac surgery can offer real value to the patients, be it cosmetic, psychological (no scar in the front), biological (less bleeding, less pain, less sternum deformity without division of the manubrium), or even sociocultural (as in some Middle Eastern countries, in which a frontal scar in female patients is considered as a doom). However, these techniques have had particular application in congenital cardiac surgery when compared with adults.

It is true that MICS in this context is mostly about minimally invasive incisions, while real minimally invasive procedures which avoid utilization of cardiopulmonary bypass are under evaluation nowadays. For the surgical approach, CPB-assisted operations with minimal thoracotomies or "hybrid procedures" have been described.

Nowadays, ASD can usually be closed by an interventional cardiologist, unless morphological features are unfavorable. This can be called a true minimally invasive method since no incision and, mostly, no CPB is involved in the procedure. It is, in fact, CPB that is more invasive since it can trigger the so-called systemic inflammatory syndrome, which is proportional to the CPB time and inversely proportional to BSA [50]. Any other attempt is rather "minimal access" surgery. However, surgery does not require X-ray exposure and allows complete repair using biological or physiological materials such as autologous or heterologous pericardium. On the contrary, current transcatheter procedures require prolonged X-ray exposure [51], and septal defect closure devices are made of a rigid metal material that is bound to stay inside the heart forever: is this going to be safe forever? Some authors have reported late device dislocation and higher risk late reoperation [5]: is this acceptable for ASD?

On the other side, Butera et al. [2] reported that ASD closure by percutaneous approach has a significantly lower rate of either total or major early post-procedural complications than surgery. However, costs remain high, and financial issues are a matter of concern in many countries with public health system. During the last few years, with increasing experience, we have observed a significant reduction in the operative times without increased risk, when compared with conventional surgery [16]. The median cost for treatment of ASDS was 7275 euros (IQR 6975-7515 euros). According to scatterplot analysis, we showed a progressive reduction of hospital costs over time ($P = 0.009$) (**Figure 11**).

In the light of our results, we are now extending our minimally invasive approaches to CHD which are more complex than ASD. Besides, the safety of the peripheral CPB convinced us to employ it progressively to lower body weight patients. We believe that soon, due to the miniaturization of surgical instruments, cannulas, and tubing systems, we will spread the use of minimally invasive surgery with peripheral CPB in even smaller children.

Since many years, it has been our institutional policy to promote a gender-differentiated minimally invasive approach for patients with CHD [52]. This has proven to be safe, and it offers excellent clinical results comparable to classic more invasive methods. In addition, in our experience, we have demonstrated a 95% patient satisfaction after RAMT, with no evidence of scoliosis, restriction to shoulder movement, breast development, or lactation problems at follow-up [15]. The only complication we could outline in our female patients with mini-thoracotomy (MT) was a temporary trivial neuro-sensorial deficit at the mammary area that disappeared in all within 6 months after surgery. In addition to the benefit of a limited cutaneous incision, a careful and gentle muscle plane dissection and reconstruction is certainly related to the high quality of our results. It is highly advisable that the MT incision be located very low in the submammary area, usually at least 4–5 cm under the right nipple and away from any possibility of future breast development.

The RALMT has been added relatively recently in our minimally invasive surgical armamentarium [45], and it has rapidly gained affidability as it has proven to be an effective and safe approach to correct patients with PAPVD from the right lung (which is even easier to identify from this approach). Also, it allows excellent visualization of the aortic root when needed (i.e., aortic cross-clamping or access to the aortic valve or sub-valvar area).

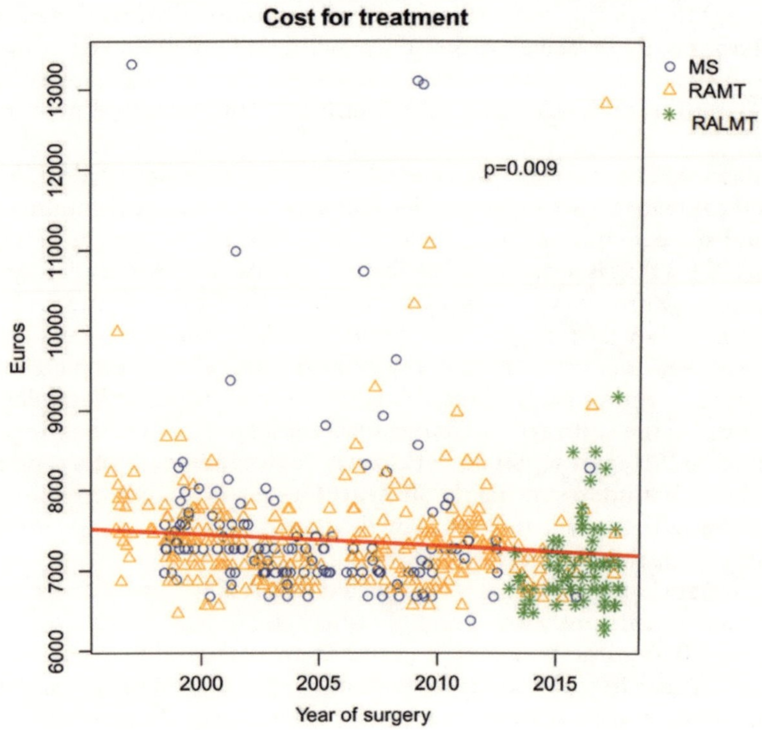

Figure 11.
Scatterplot showing the variation of the overall cost of treatment for surgical ostium secundum atrial septal defect closure, by year of surgery. MS, mini-sternotomy; RAMT, right anterior mini-thoracotomy; RALMT, right lateral mini-thoracotomy (modified from Vida et al. [16]).

In our two decades of experience, induced ventricular fibrillation has been a safe and reproducible technique, which we have always associated with mild systemic protective hypothermia [7, 25, 26]. It avoids cumbersome cross-clamping and consequently allows smaller access especially in RAMT or RALMT approaches. Nonetheless, we are also aware that a cross-clamping through RAMT can also be used when needed [28]. With the recent introduction of the RALMT, which exposes the ascending aorta much better, aortic cross-clamping can be quickly done employing a Novare Straight Cygnus Aortic Cross Clamp in adults or even with conventional Chitwood clamps in children.

Intraoperative TEE echocardiographic monitoring is of paramount importance in such limited surgical exposure since it can ensure a total de-airing of the left chambers together with a complete assessment of the surgical correction and detection of possible residual lesions. Furthermore, the utilization of Trendelenburg position as a default position during open heart surgery on induced FV is a new safety strategy to prevent a cerebral air embolism.

The use of a peripheral CPB has been shown to be a safe and excellent option in selected patients [18, 19], since it permits minimal surgical incisions, consequently reducing the patient's surgical trauma. As mentioned above, the NIRS monitoring of the blood perfusion to the lower extremities in patients with peripheral CPB is a useful tool to control blood flow perfusion variations to the lower extremities during CPB time. It is of notice that we were never required to convert peripheral to central CPB because of issues with lower limb blood flow. However, critical NIRS levels (<30%) has been reached in patients with a bodyweight of less than 15 kg for a maximum period of 30 min, which has entirely normalized after arterial decannulation as did the postoperative myoglobin and creatine phosphokinase levels (within 12 hours). Last, we needed to patch repair the femoral artery only in five patients among all. However, as we shifted to the subaxillary (muscle sparse) approach, we have switched to central aortic cannulation utilizing the same arterial cannula (Medtronic Bio-Medicus NextGen MN, USA), to avoid residual stenosis in borderline femoral arteries (in children < than 15 kg).

6. Conclusions

Minimally invasive cardiac surgery for CHD consists in the minimization of surgical access with consequent reduction of surgical trauma, reduced postoperative pain, and a more prompt recovery that can permit a decrease in hospital stays and costs. Despite minimal incisions, in our hands, these techniques have allowed optimal repair which is comparable to the conventional surgery ones in terms of safety, with an additional better cosmetic result and a better-perceived quality of the treatment by the patients, especially female, with less psychological discomfort caused by the more traditional sternal scars. The technological advancement (such as vacuum-assisted venous drainage, new retracting systems, and the use of peripheral cannulation for CPB) has permitted further miniaturization of our incisions without increasing patients' morbidity and, on the contrary, improving results and patients' satisfaction. The recent lateralization of surgical access has added another benefit contributing to an increase in the types of CHD we can treat, with no additional risk. Nowadays, MICS for CHD continues to evolve and expand with growing technology and surgeon experience. It is safe and effective for various types of CHD, and it does not appear to result in significant differences in short-term and long-term survival and freedom from adverse events when compared with the more traditional midline sternotomy approaches. It seems to result in faster recovery to healthy routine life, reducing the length of hospital stay and better satisfaction among patents. As this compares favorably with percutaneous techniques, MICS for CHD is now to be considered the gold standard for surgical repair of simple and moderately severe CHD which are not amenable or borderline for transcatheter repair.

Acknowledgements

We acknowledge Mr. Nicola Paccagnella (Department of Cardiac, Thoracic, Vascular Sciences and Public Health, University of Padova Medical School, Italy) for the artwork. We had no fundings.

Conflict of interest

The authors declare no conflict of interest.

Acronyms

CHD	congenital heart disease
LPEMT	left posterior extrapleuric mini-thoracotomy
MICS	minimally invasive cardiac surgery
MS	midline mini-sternotomy

RAMT	right anterior mini-thoracotomy
RALMT	right axillary lateral mini-thoracotomy
RPMT	right posterior mini-thoracotomy

Author details

Massimo A. Padalino*, Demetrio G. Pittarello, Vladimiro L. Vida and Giovanni Stellin
Department of Cardiac, Thoracic, Vascular Sciences and Public Health, University of Padova Medical School, Italy

*Address all correspondence to: massimo.padalino@unipd.it

References

[1] Lewis FJ, Varco RL, Taufic M. Repair of atrial septal defects in man under direct vision with the aid of hypothermia. Surgery. 1954;**36**:538-556

[2] Butera G, De Rosa G, Chessa M, Rosti L, Negura DG, Luciane P, et al. Transcatheter closure of atrial septal defect in young children: Results and follow-up. Journal of the American College of Cardiology. 2003;**42**:241-245

[3] Thomson JD, Aburawi EH, Watterson KG, Van Doorn C, Gibbs JL. Surgical and transcatheter (Amplatzer) closure of atrial septal defects: A prospective comparison of results and cost. Heart. 2002;**87**:466-469

[4] Sarris GE, Kirvassilis G, Zavaropoulos P, Belli E, Berggren H, Carrel T, et al. Surgery for complications of transcatheter closure of atrial septal defects: A multi-institutional study from the European congenital heart surgeons association. European Journal of Cardio-Thoracic Surgery. 2010;**37**:1285-1290

[5] del Nido PJ. Minimal incision congenital cardiac surgery. Seminars in Thoracic and Cardiovascular Surgery. 2007;**19**:319-324

[6] Cremer JT, Boning A, Anssar MB, Kim PY, Pethig K, Harringer W, et al. Different approaches for minimally invasive closure of atrial septal defects. The Annals of Thoracic Surgery. 1999;**67**:1648-1652

[7] Nicholson IA, Bichell DP, Bacha EA, del Nido PJ. Minimal sternotomy approach for congenital heart operations. The Annals of Thoracic Surgery. 2001;**71**:469-472

[8] Kadner A, Dodge-Khatami A, Dave H, Knirsch W, Bettex D, Pretre R. Closure of restrictive ventricular septal defects through a right axillary thoracotomy. The Heart Surgery Forum. 2006;**9**:E836-E839

[9] Mishaly D, Ghosh P, Preisman S. Minimally invasive congenital cardiac surgery through right anterior minithoracotomy approach. The Annals of Thoracic Surgery. 2008;**85**:831-835

[10] Grinda JM, Folliguet TA, Dervanian P, Mace L, Legault B, Neveux JY. Right anterolateral thoracotomy for repair of atrial septal defect. The Annals of Thoracic Surgery. 1996;**62**:175-178

[11] Yoshimura N, Yamaguchi M, Oshima Y, Oka S, Ootaki Y, Yoshida M. Repair of atrial septal defect through a right posterolateral thoracotomy: A cosmetic approach for female patients. The Annals of Thoracic Surgery. 2001;**72**:2103-2105

[12] Houyel L, Petit J, Planche C, Sousa-Uva M, Roussin R, Belli E, et al. Right postero-lateral thoracotomy for open heart surgery in infants and children. Indications and results. Archives des Maladies du Coeur et des Vaisseaux. 1999;**92**:641-646

[13] Metras D, Kreitmann B. Correction of cardiac defects through a right thoracotomy in children. The Journal of Thoracic and Cardiovascular Surgery. 1999;**117**:1040-1042

[14] Bleiziffer S, Schreiber C, Burgkart R, Regenfelder F, Kostolny M, Libera P, et al. The influence of right anterolateral thoracotomy in prepubescent female patients on late breast development and on the incidence of scoliosis. The Journal of Thoracic and Cardiovascular Surgery. 2004;**127**:1474-1480

[15] Vida VL, Tessari C, Fabozzo A, Padalino MA, Barzon E, Zucchetta F, et al. The evolution of the right

anterolateral thoracotomy technique for correction of atrial septal defects: Cosmetic and functional results in prepubescent patients. The Annals of Thoracic Surgery. 2013;**95**:242-247

[16] Vida VL, Zanotto L, Zanotto L, Tessari C, Padalino MA, Zanella F, et al. Minimally invasive surgery for atrial septal defects: A 20-year experience at a single centre. Interactive Cardiovascular and Thoracic Surgery. 2019;**28**:961-967. DOI: 10.1093/icvts/ivz017

[17] Matsumoto M, Oka Y, Strom J, Frishman W, Kadish A, Becker RM, et al. Application of transesophageal echocardiography to continuous intraoperative monitoring of left ventricular performance. The American Journal of Cardiology. 1980;**46**:95-105

[18] Shanewise JS, Cheung AT, Aronson S, Stewart WJ, Weiss RL, Mark JB, et al. ASE/SCA guidelines for performing a comprehensive intraoperative multiplane transesophageal echocardiography examination: Recommendations of the American Society of Echocardiography Council for intraoperative echocardiography and the Society of Cardiovascular Anesthesiologists Task Force for certification in perioperative transesophageal echocardiography. Journal of the American Society of Echocardiography. 1999;**12**:884-900

[19] Stokes JW. Transoesophageal echocardiography in routine cardiac surgery. The Medical Journal of Australia. 2005;**182**:93-94

[20] Ayres NA, Miller-Hance W, Fyfe DA, Stevenson JG, Sahn DJ, Young LT, et al. Indications and guidelines for performance of transesophageal echocardiography in the patient with pediatric acquired or congenital heart disease: Report from the task force of the Pediatric Council of the American Society of echocardiography. Journal of the American Society of Echocardiography. 2005;**18**:91-98

[21] Sheil ML, Baines DB. Intraoperative transoesophageal echocardiography for paediatric cardiac surgery-an audit of 200 cases. Anaesthesia and Intensive Care. 1999;**27**:591-595

[22] Fanshawe M, Ellis C, Habib S, Konstadt SN, Reich DL. A retrospective analysis of the costs and benefits related to alterations in cardiac surgery from routine intraoperative transesophageal echocardiography. Anesthésie et Analgésie. 2002;**95**:824-827

[23] Ramamoorthy C, Lynn AM, Stevenson JG. Pro: Transesophageal echocardiography should be routinely used during pediatric open cardiac surgery. Journal of Cardiothoracic and Vascular Anesthesia. 1999;**13**:629-631

[24] Kamra K, Russell I, Miller-Hance WC. Role of transesophageal echocardiography in the management of pediatric patients with congenital heart disease. Pediatric Anesthesia. 2011;**21**:479-493

[25] Jijeh AMZ, Omran AS, Najm HK, Abu-Sulaiman RM. Role of intraoperative transesophageal echocardiography in pediatric cardiac surgery. Journal of the Saudi Heart Association. 2016;**28**:89-94

[26] Muhiudeen IA, Roberson DA, Silverman NH, Haas GS, Turley K, Cahalan MK. Intraoperative echocardiography for evaluation of congenital heart defects in infants and children. Anesthesiology. 1992;**76**:165-172

[27] Scohy TV, Matte G, van Neer PL, van der Steen AF, McGhie J, Bogers A, et al. A new transesophageal probe for newborns. Ultrasound in Medicine & Biology. 2009;**35**:1686-1689

[28] Scohy TV, Gommers D, Schepp MN, Gommers D, Schepp MN, McGhie J,

et al. Image quality using a micromultiplane transesophageal echocardiographic probe in older children during cardiac surgery. European Journal of Anaesthesiology. 2009;**26**:445-447

[29] Ma XJ, Huang GY, Liang XC, Chen ZG, Jia B, Li X, et al. Transoesophageal echocardiography in monitoring, guiding, and evaluating surgical repair of congenital cardiac malformations in children. Cardiology in the Young. 2007;**17**:301-306

[30] Balmer C, Barron D, Wright JG, de Giovanni JV, Miller P, Dhillon R, et al. Experience with intraoperative ultrasound in paediatric cardiac surgery. Cardiology in the Young. 2006;**16**:455-462

[31] Aronson LA. Trans-nasal placement of biplane transesophageal echocardiography probe intraoperatively in an adolescent with congenital heart disease. Anesthesia and Analgesia. 2003;**97**:1617-1619

[32] Rice MJ, McDonald RW, Li X, Shen I, Ungerleider RM, Sahn DJ. New technology and methodologies for intraoperative, perioperative, and intraprocedural monitoring of surgical and catheter interventions for congenital heart disease. Echocardiography. 2002;**19**:725-734

[33] Bruce CJ, O'Leary P, Hagler DJ, Seward JB, Cabalka AK. Miniaturized transesophageal echocardiography in newborn infants. Journal of the American Society of Echocardiography. 2002;**15**:791-797

[34] Lake CL. Fast-tracking in paediatric cardiac anesthesia: An update. Annals of Cardiac Anaesthesia. 2002;**5**:203-206

[35] Laussen P, Roth S. Fast tracking: Efficiently and safely moving patients through the intensive care unit. Progress in Pediatric Cardiology. 2003;**18**:149-158

[36] Metin K, Celik M, Oto O. Fast-track anesthesia in cardiac surgery for noncomplex congenital cardiac anomalies. Pediatrics and Neonatology. 2005;**5**:2

[37] Mittnacht AJC, Thanjan M, Srivastava S, Joashi U, Bodian C, Hossain S, et al. Extubation in the operating room after congenital heart surgery in children. The Journal of Thoracic and Cardiovascular Surgery. 2008;**136**:88-93

[38] Demetrio P, Shafer K. Anesthesia for minimally invasive cardiac surgery. In: Vida V, Stellin G, editors. Fundamentals of Congenital Minimally Invasive Cardiac Surgery. USA: Elsevier; 2018

[39] Vogt A, Stieger DS, Theurillat C, Curatolo M. Single-injection thoracic paravertebral block for postoperative pain treatment after thoracoscopic surgery. British Journal of Anaesthesia. 2005;**95**:816-821

[40] Nagahiro I, Andou A, Aoe M, Sano Y, Date H, Shimizu N. Pulmonary function, postoperative pain, and serum cytokine level after lobectomy: A comparison of VATS and conventional procedure. The Annals of Thoracic Surgery. 2001;**72**:362-365

[41] Karmakar MK. Thoracic paravertebral block. Anesthesiology. 2001;**95**:771-780

[42] Jamieson BD, Mariano ER. Thoracic and lumbar paravertebral blocks for outpatient lithotripsy. Journal of Clinical Anesthesia. 2007;**19**:149-151

[43] Sabanathan S, Smith PJ, Pradhan GN, Hashimi H, Eng JB, Mearns AJ. Continuous intercostal nerve block for pain relief after thoracotomy. The Annals of Thoracic Surgery. 1988;**46**:425-426

[44] Myles PS, Bain C. Underutilization of paravertebral block in thoracic

surgery. Journal of Cardiothoracic and Vascular Anesthesia. 2006;**20**:635-638

[45] Vida VL, Padalino MA, Motta R, Stellin G. Minimally invasive surgical options in pediatric heart surgery. Expert Review of Cardiovascular Therapy. 2011;**9**(6):763-769. DOI: 10.1586/erc.11.69. Review

[46] Vida VL, Tiberio I, Gallo M, Guariento A, Suti E, Pittarello D, et al. Percutaneous internal jugular venous cannulation for extracorporeal circulation during minimally invasive technique in children with congenital heart disease: Operative technique and results. Minerva Pediatrica. 2016;**68**:341-347

[47] Vida VL, Tessari C, Putzu A, Tiberio I, Guariento A, Gallo M, et al. The peripheral cannulation technique in minimally invasive congenital cardiac surgery. The International Journal of Artificial Organs. 2016;**39**:300-303. DOI: 10.5301/ijao.5000505

[48] Vida VL, Padalino MA, Boccuzzo G, Stellin G. Near-infrared spectroscopy for monitoring leg perfusion during minimally invasive surgery for patients with congenital heart defects. The Journal of Thoracic and Cardiovascular Surgery. 2012;**143**:756-757

[49] Speggiorin S, Padalino MA, Vida VL, Bonato R, Stellin G. Cardiac herniation. After minimally invasive cardiac surgery: An unusual potentially lethal complication. Circulation. 2009;**120**: 2509-2510

[50] Leon-Wyss J, Vida VL, Veras O, Vides I, Gaitan G, O'Connell M, et al. Modified extrapleural ligation of patent ductus arteriosus: A convenient surgical approach in a developing country. The Annals of Thoracic Surgery. 2005;**79**:632-635

[51] Vida VL, Rubino M, Bottio T, Padalino MA, Milanesi O, Pittarello D, et al. Thoracoscopic closure of the patent arterial duct. Cardiology in the Young. 2004;**14**:164-167

[52] Vida VL, Padalino MA, Boccuzzo G, Veshti AA, Speggiorin S, Falasco G, et al. Minimally invasive operation for congenital heart disease: A sex-differentiated approach. The Journal of Thoracic and Cardiovascular Surgery. 2009;**138**:933-936

Chapter 7

Revascularisation Strategies in OPCAB (Off Pump Coronary Artery Bypass)

Murali P. Vettath, Kannan A. Vellachamy, Nitin Ganagadharan, Madhu Ravisankar, Smera Koroth and Gopalakrishnan Raman

Abstract

OPCAB was performed before the advent of heart lung machine. But with the development of stabilizers, coronary artery bypass grafting has been performed over the last two decades successfully in many centres around the world. But still 80% of bypass surgeries are done on the heart lung machine. We were one of the few teams who have been performing this OPCAB for the past 18 years. All along, we have been innovating, fabricating and developing and patenting instruments, techniques and technology to help us perform OPCAB in 100% of all our coronary patients. That too being able to reduce the mortality of bypass surgery to less than 0.5%. In this chapter, we have attempted to write down our strategy, in order to successfully perform OPCAB in all our patients, so that the coming generation can benefit from it.

Keywords: OPCAB, CABG, arterial graft, venous graft, bilateral mammary grafting, IABP, mammary patch, VAO, SIMS, stabilizer

1. Introduction

OPCAB has been the procedure of choice in quite a few centres around the world. Though, the numbers of surgeons performing 100% of their CABGs off pump are still miniscule. The main issue is that performing OPCAB in all patients becomes quite strenuous for some surgeons because in OPCAB, the margin of error is very low. And that when a patient is converted to the heart lung machine then the morbidity and the mortality is high. The learning curve is very steep in order to master this technique. Our team had to perform over 500 OPCABs till the team became comfortable to perform this procedure in all patients who needed coronary revascularisation. There are two important issues that have to be tackled before a team gets to be able to perform 100% OPCABs over a decade [1]. One is the mind set and another is team work. If one achieves these two goals, then the rest is only a question of time, when the team could achieve it. Every team player has to become confident that we would be able re-vascularise every patient without going on pump. That confidence and strategy is the key to the success of the surgery. Apart from preparing for surgery, and planning for difficult cases, the execution,

IntechOpen

intraoperative and post-operative management till he returns to his room and to his further follow up, all are to be planned and executed with precision. Every patient needs to get a tailor made surgical approach. As, no two coronaries are same. Likewise no two grafting are same. Accordingly no two patients would have same postoperative course. Hence there should be no slackness on the part of the team thinking that it is just a straight forward case and we can relax. We have always found that we make mistakes when we are not agile or when we take things for granted. As every patient is important. Hence, we should care for him like we care for our parents or our colleague. Once we are able to achieve this, then success can be assured.

2. Surgical strategy

In this chapter, we would like to present our view on how we plan our surgical strategy. Starting from the type of surgery, which the patient is going to undergo, to the revascularisation techniques which we plan are going to be discussed here. As we said, every patient needs to have his surgery tailor made according to his specific needs. Our main aim is to perform complete revascularisation on all patients, then, the next priority is to perform the coronary bypass without using the heart lung machine. Then our priority is to use arterial grafts where ever possible. The use of left internal mammary artery (LIMA) to the left anterior descending artery (LAD) is a rule or standard for all patients. We have noticed that as the LAD is the most important artery in the heart, if the LIMA remains patent over 10 years then it usually remains open for life [2]. The presence of nitric oxide in LIMA in fact does not allow any clot formation inside it and that even a small LIMA remains patent as long as the run off of the LAD is good. And that once we anastomose a LIMA to the LAD, then it is unlikely that the LAD distal to the anastomosis would develop atherosclerosis. This is because of the nitric oxide that is secreted from the LIMA which prevents the development of atherosclerosis being formed in that region. This is unlike in case of drug eluting stent where we see narrowing of the vessel distal to the stent.

3. Preoperative preparation in OPCAB

Preparation of patients in OPCAB is rather less cumbersome than in patients with on-pump CABG. That is, we do not have to stop the antiplatelet medication in patients who are going to undergo OPCAB. Hence in patients with acute coronary syndrome we have the advantage of continuing the antiplatelet and the injection heparin till the day of surgery. Thereby avoiding ischemia in these patients. The only medicine we stop is beta blockers on the day of surgery. As we do not wish to reduce the heart rates unlike in other centres, we in fact like to increase the heart rate so as to increase the cardiac output in turn. This is how we are able to avoid the use of inotropes in all our patients during the positioning of the heart before grafting [1]. Apart from this there are no changes in the management of patients in either groups.

4. Anaesthesia management

Anaesthetic management of patient being induced for OPCAB is similar in line, as for all cardiac surgical patients, except that they are not totally ironed out.

This is to make sure that the mean blood pressure is maintained above 75 mm of Hg, all through the procedure, though this warrants a separate chapter.

5. Surgical techniques in OPCAB

5.1 Harvesting of the conduit

Once the patient is positioned, painted and draped (**Figures 1** and **2**).

The idea is to harvest the arterial grafts first and then the vein graft if necessary. The skin incision extends from 2 cm below the sternal notch to 1 cm above the xiphoid process. We usually dissect the xiphoid process out from both sides and its attachment below from the diaphragm using diathermy (which is at 70 coagulation and zero on the cutting—that is our setting on the diathermy). Hence the sternotomy starts by cutting the xiphoid out first and then starting the sternotomy as usual. The chest is opened as usual and the pericardium is slit longitudinally to expose the heart. The pericardium near the diaphragm is cut along the diaphragm up to the inferior vena cava (IVC). This is done after the right pleura is opened and the thymus is tied up near the superior vena cava (SVC). This helps in allowing the heart to lie freely when the heart is being positioned during grafting of the lateral wall vessels.

It is very important to maintain strict haemostasis all through the opening of the sternum till grafting at least—as all these patients are on antiplatelet medications and/or on heparin, so any bleeding site left unattended at this stage would cause unnecessary blood loss (photo of chest opened before harvesting the mammary). Hence, if we spend time for haemostasis during opening of the chest, then the closing becomes easy and tidy.

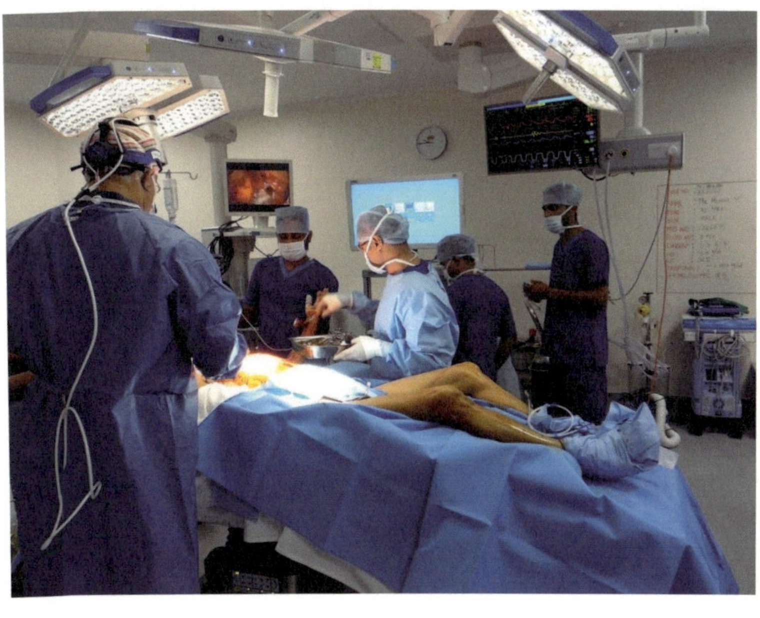

Figure 1.
Patient on the table with left arm on the side for radial artery harvesting.

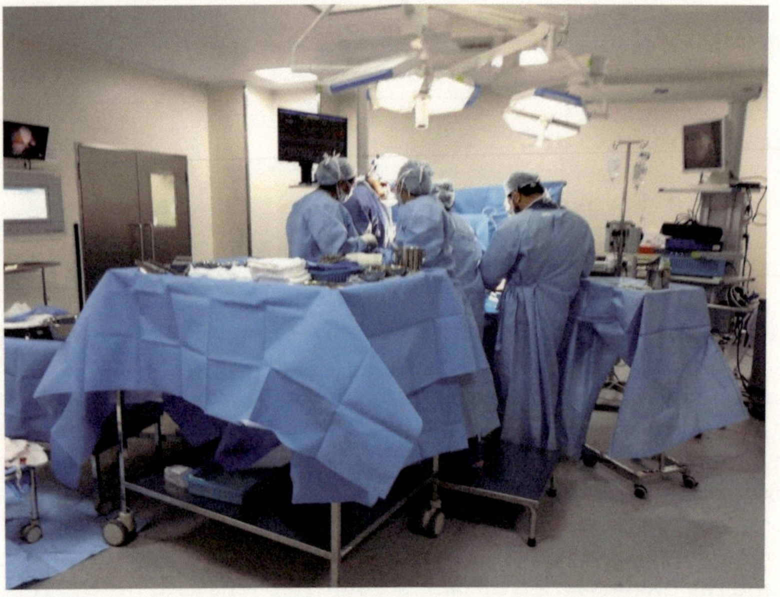

Figure 2.
Shows the patient after draping and the surgery in progress, with chest being opened and the radial artery being harvested simultaneously.

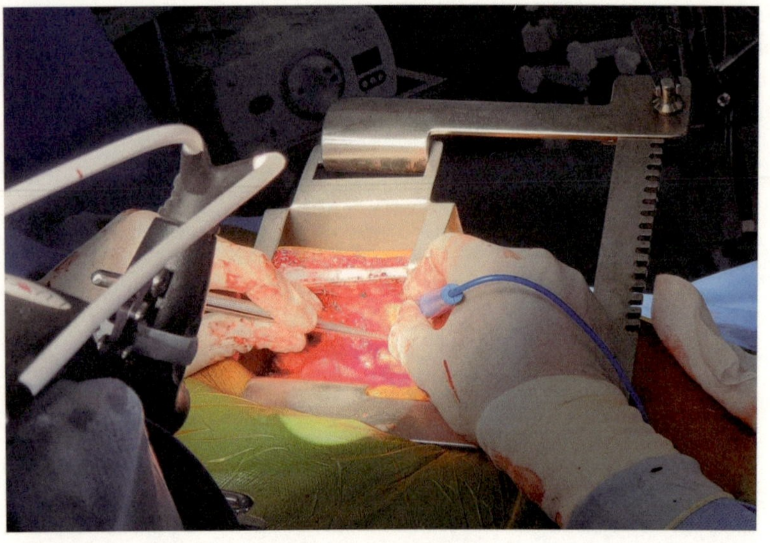

Figure 3.
Shows the IMA retractor in position.

5.2 Harvesting the LIMA

The internal mammary artery (IMA) of the left side is the most important artery and that we need to harvest it with caution. And it is important to maintain hemodynamic all through this dissection, so that we can do a good job, as it is important to remember that the patient's longevity depends on the patency of LIMA anastomosis being patent all through. Earlier we used to dissect the LIMA as a pedicle, but for the last 2 years we have mastered this technique of Skeletonised mammary dissection, with a cold cautery technique, which does not allow the

LIMA to go into spasm during the harvesting. The cautery is usually set at 40 coagulation and no cutting during the mammary harvesting. The blood pressure is maintained at a systolic blood pressure between 130 and 140 mm during the dissection, so that we have a good pressure head and the mammary pulsates during the dissection.

After the lift sternum is lifted (IMA retractor in position **Figure 3**).

The left pleura is opened longitudinally parallel to the sternum up to the top, after the branches crossing it are clipped and cut with a forehand scissors. The LIMA dissection starts from the xiphoid region. The Thoracic fascia is dissected using the diathermy by making a parallel incision on it medial to the LIMA all along the sternal edge. Then the cautery tip is now used as a cold cautery for all the dissections from now on. The tip is used to dissect the LIMA away from the thoracic fascia by moving the tip upward towards the LIMA and then used the tip on the diathermy to push the tissues up and away from the LIMA again, pushing the LIMA down from the chest wall to expose the intercostal branches, would cause avulsion of these branches at its base, which would end up in dissection of the LIMA. Once the distal end is dissected at the LIMA bifurcation, the two branches are clipped using two clips on the distal end and one liga clip on the proximal end, and then cutting it with the forward cutting Castroviejo scissors. At this stage no heparin is given. Dilute injection Papaverine is sprayed on the dissected end and the dissection is continued all through till the first branch of LIMA (LIMA dissection **Figure 4**).

In fact the IMA does not clot as its wall exudes nitric oxide and because it is clipped at the end and the blood pressure is maintained above 130 mm systolic it gets bigger by the time the dissection is over. The video of skeletonised LIMA is seen in the following link; SKELTONISED LIMA DISSECTION USING COLD CAUTERY TECHNIQUE. https://youtu.be/m7mYWLQsDAE.

Once LIMA is dissected, then RIMA is also dissected depending on the revascularisation strategy.

Simultaneously, the radial artery from the left hand is harvested. This is also taken down as a skeletonised artery and it is dilated with injection papaverine, which is injected intraluminally and clipped at end and stored in warm heparinised saline in a bowl. The important point to make sure in patients whose radial artery is harvested is to make sure that the pulse-oxymeter saturation of the thumb should always show the wave form and that it should be 100% at any given time. The arm has to be closed only after perfect haemostasis, and to make sure that the

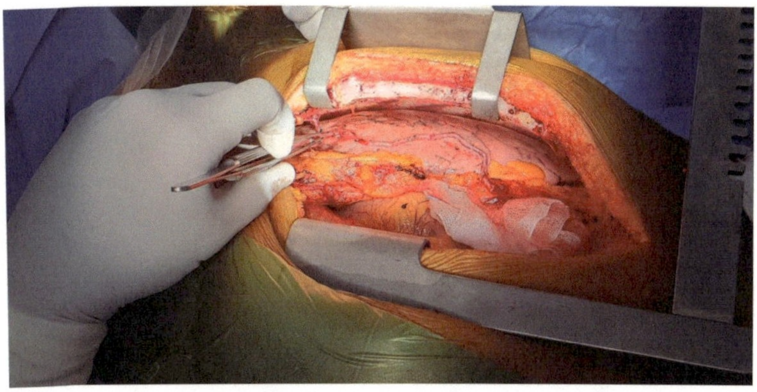

Figure 4.
Shows skeletonised LIMA after dissection.

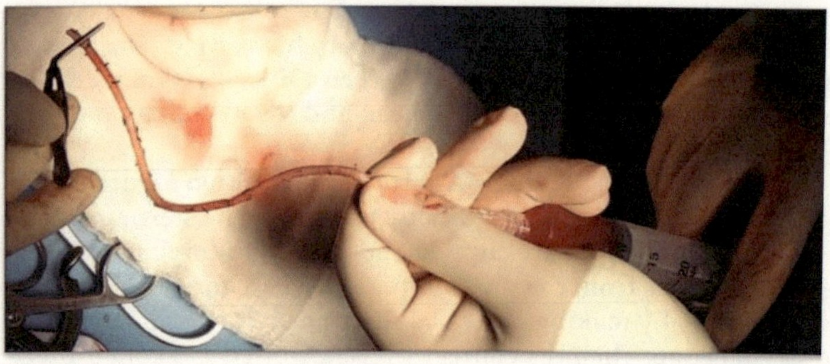

Figure 5.
Showing skeletonised radial artery.

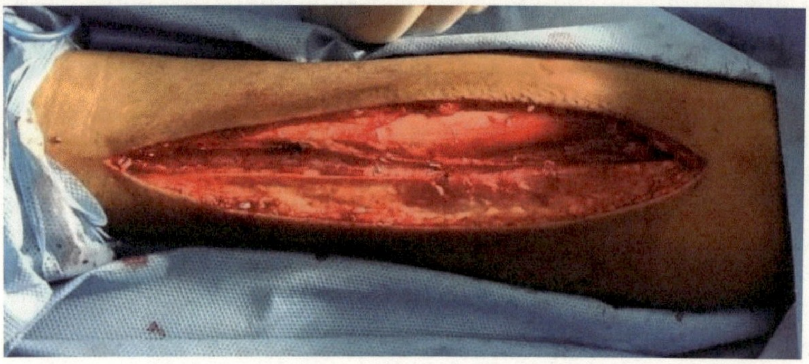

Figure 6.
Showing the haemostasis in the forearm after the radial artery is harvested.

crepe bandage applied is not too tight. We do not use any specific vasodilators like nitroglycerin or post-operative Diltiazem, as we make sure that the Radial artery is grafted only on coronaries with more than 80% lesions for sure (**Figure 5**, showing the skeletonised radial artery) (**Figure 6**).

The radial artery dissection video is seen in the following link: https://youtu.be/19YY37hpeTs—radial artery dissection.

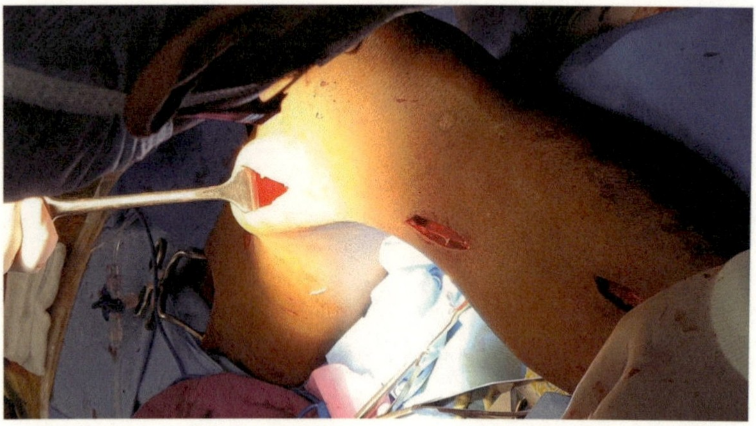

Figure 7.
Showing the skip technique of SVG being harvested.

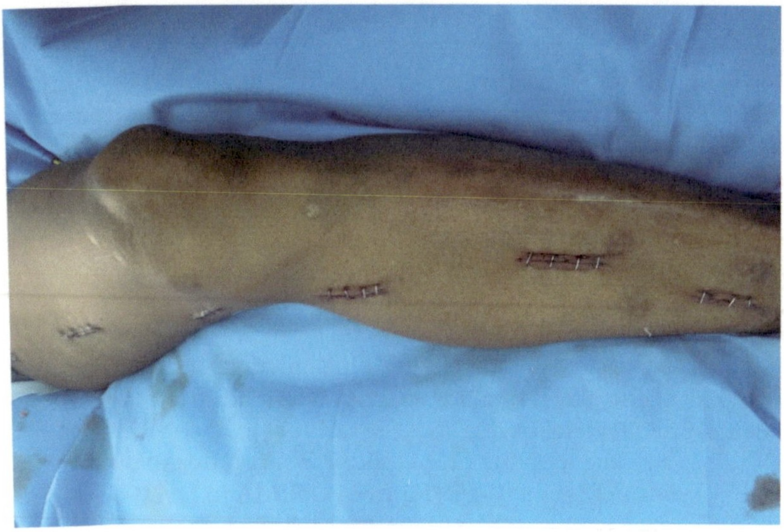

Figure 8.
Showing the skip incisions on the lower limb after closing with clips.

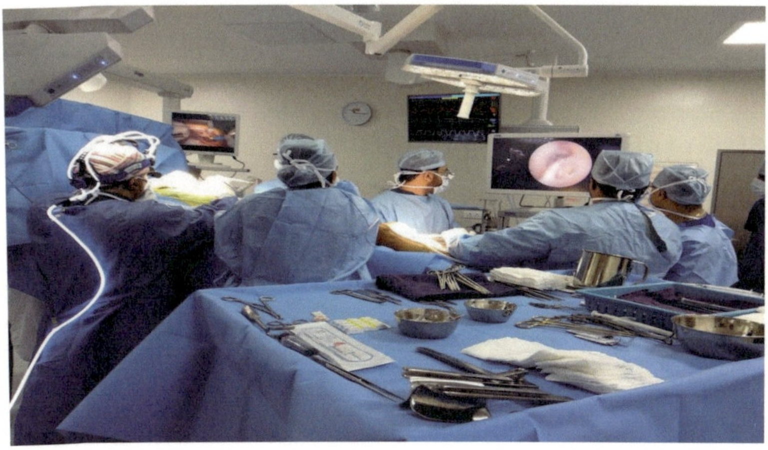

Figure 9.
Showing EVH being done.

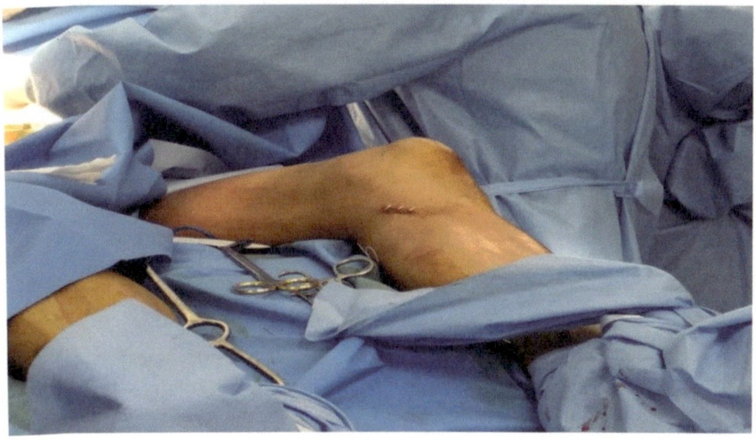

Figure 10.
Showing the single small scar after EVH technique... but this comes with a cost.

The third conduit that is harvested is usually the long saphenous vein (SVG). It is either harvested from the thigh or from the leg. It is dissected as an open technique or by a skip technique (**Figures 7** and **8**), showing the skip technique of SVG being harvested (avoiding a continuous incision and the wound afterward) which does not need any extra instrumentation.

The other technique is to use endoscopic vein harvesting technique (EVH) **Figures 9** and **10**.

5.3 Grafting sequence

The first artery to be grafted is usually the LAD (left anterior descending), and always by LIMA unless there is an issue. This is the link that shows our grafting pattern.

The video link of the play list is: https://www.youtube.com/playlist?list=PLmvb6npEfabinhlatq8IYLBz8WlHo8bu1.

In case there is an issue with the LIMA, like it is short, due to dissection or injury, either we use the R(right)IMA (**Figure 11**, RIMA to LAD) or the radial artery or the vein piece hocked to the LIMA to reach the LAD.

This link shows: LIMA TO RADIAL ANASTAMOSED TO LAD, DIAGONAL AND MARG CIRC as a 'C' graft: https://youtu.be/OaOjXlRk7Nk.

Sometimes when we use RIMA to LAD, if it is long enough, then we use LIMA to radial and skip to all the coronaries. If we plan for a total arterial grafting, the preference is to have two inflows to the coronaries if both the left and the right coronary artery need grafting. But if it is only the left system that need grafting and if we plan for a total arterial grafting with no touch technique of the aorta, then LIMA—RIMA Y or LIMA—radial Y is used.

Video links showing:

BIMA-LIMA TO DIAGONAL AND LAD. RIMA TO RADIAL SKIP TO PDA AND PLV: https://youtu.be/96LLBz1hS5k.

BIMA-LIMA TO DIAGONAL-LAD.RIMA TO RADIAL SKIP TO RAMOS, OM & PDA: https://youtu.be/fJ_kLZmQV6I.

BIMA-LIMA TO DIAGONAL AND LAD. RIMA TO RADIAL SKIP TO OM & PDA: https://youtu.be/SN1F8YjPiUA

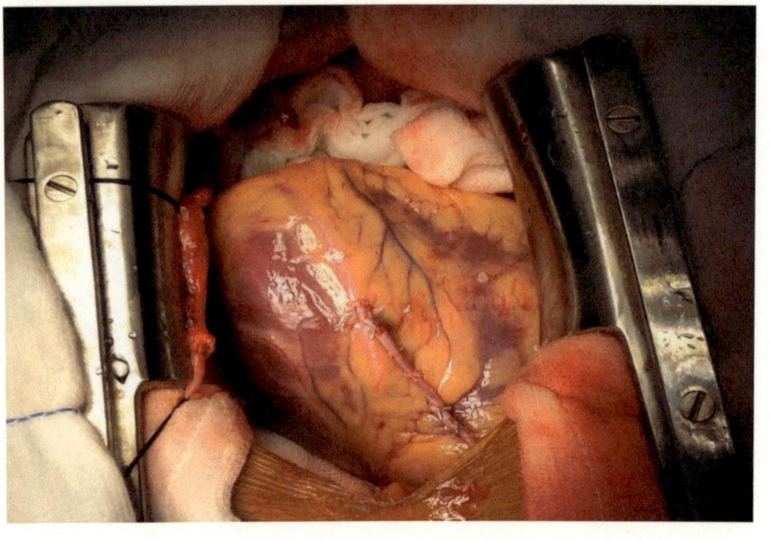

Figure 11.
Shows RIMA anastomosed to LAD.

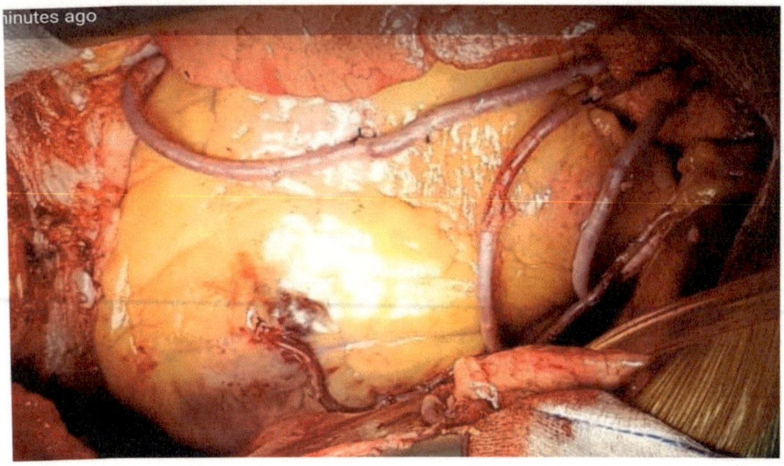

Figure 12.
Shows the usual OPCAB × 5 (LIMA to diagonal skip to LAD and SVG to OM1, OM2 and PDA).

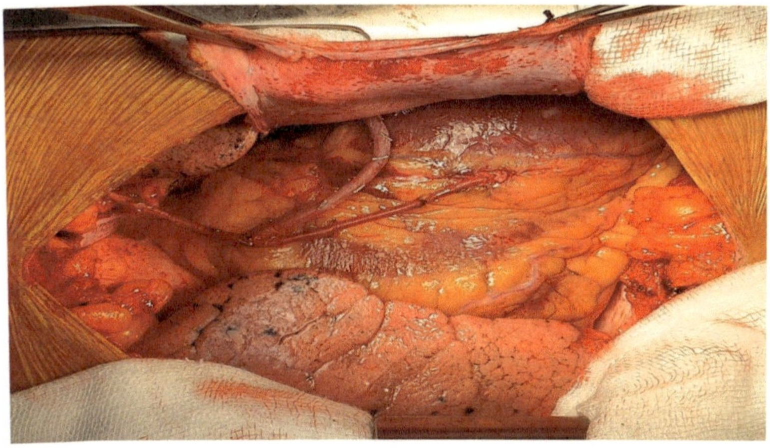

Figure 13.
Shows LIMA—radial Y graft.

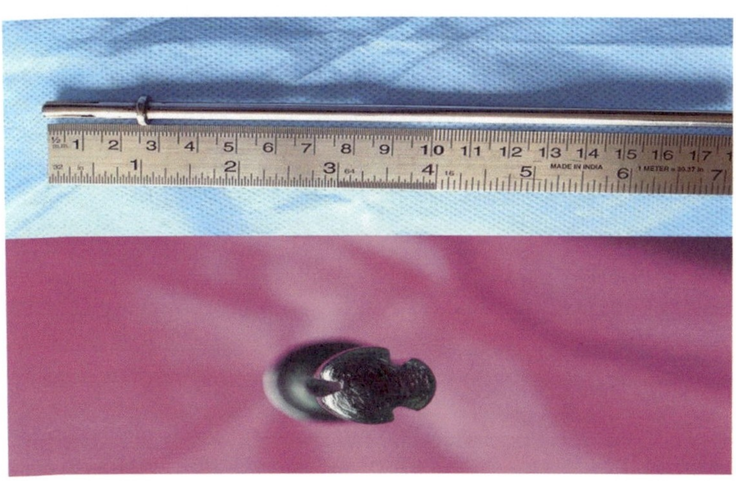

Figure 14.
Shows the VAO (Vettath's anastomotic obturator).

BIMA and radial. LIMA TO LAD, LIMA-RADIAL TO DIAGONAL, RIMA TO RADIAL TO PDA: https://youtu.be/sWa2N3qlCm4.

Most of the elderly patients (above 75–80 years of age) we stick to LIMA and vein grafts.

(**Figure 12**), or LIMA—Radial Y if only left system is involved (**Figure 13**)

The only difference is that the vein grafts are connected to the aorta without using the side clamp. In such patients who has some island of soft aortic wall left, or if they have a patch of non-calcified aorta left, we use the VAO (Vettath's anastomotic obturator) (**Figure 14**, showing the VAO).

This is one of our earliest innovations, way back in 2004, which was published in HSF [3–5]. **Figure 15**, showing the vein graft being anastomosed to the aorta using VAO.

This is the video link of the VAO being used: https://youtu.be/10eNQbPhLR0.

Because of the increasing number of diabetic patients and patients with diffusely diseased coronary arteries and with increasing amount of patients undergoing triple vessel stenting, cardiac surgeons end up getting the worst set of patients who needs a CABG. Hence, in this scenario we had developed our own technique of mammary patch on diffusely diseased LAD without endarterectomy on beating heart [6, 7].

The link of the video showing mammary patch is as follows:

https://youtu.be/bLNj2Xfjt9w Mammary Patch using Aorto Coronary Shunt.

https://youtu.be/vEQfIcsarG8 MAMMARY PATCH angioplasty using long intra coronary Shunt.

https://youtu.be/peoxcDu67m0 Long Mammary Patch angioplasty using Double Stabilizer.

It is very important to understand that when we do a mammary patch using the left IMA, then, this LIMA should never be shared with any other conduit. It should be dedicated only to the LAD.

In patients with buried coronary arteries, it is important to identify them using all the techniques we do while we are on pump, and use it in off pump. It is important to position the heart first so that it does not cause any hemodynamic compromise during stabilisation and grafting (video link as for SIMS). The LIMA stich, of putting a stay in the pericardium using a dexon stitch and lifting the pericardium

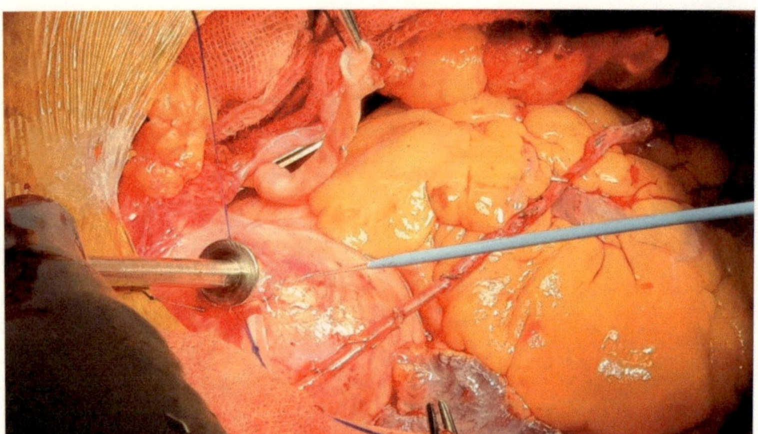

Figure 15.
Shows RIMA-radial to LAD, SVG to obtuse marginal artery, which is attached to aorta using the VAO.

to expose the lateral wall of the heart without compromising the haemodynamics is very useful to avoid conversions.

In patients who are ischaemic and unstable with big lateral wall vessels which are tightly stenosed, or in patients with dilated myocardium or huge heart, we end up using an intra-aortic balloon pump (IABP).

Usually in an ischaemic patient we notice that the ST segments go down by the time we are half way through the IMA dissection and then when the blood pressure drops, we end up putting the head end of the patient down, so as to increase the preload. When we do that, we see that the heart distends and the Pulmonary artery pressure goes up and then the patient becomes more ischaemic as his end diastolic pressure goes up and he develops sub-endocardial ischemia. In such patients irrespective of the systemic pressure its better off having the head end of the patient up, which empties the heart a bit and pulmonary artery pressure comes down and it is important to increase the heart rate so that it also helps in increasing stroke volume and the cardiac output. But in case that does not work, then we have to insert an IABP to salvage the situation. Because every patient who undergo OPCAB in our centre has two arterial lines, one in the Radial artery and another in the Femoral artery. The one in the femoral region is exchanged to an IABP using the Seldinger technique [8]. This has been a boon for us, as we are able to place the IABP immediately, and then go on with the grafting without going on the heart lung machine (HLM).

Over the last 15 years we have noticed that we were able to remove the IABP from the patient after the grafting is complete and after reversal of heparin. This innovation has worked so far and we never had to reinsert one in the ICU again on these patients (**Table 1**).

OPCAB statistics					
From	**To**	**OPCAB**	**Conversion**	**IABP removed in OT**	**Mortality no**
01-2003	12-2003	177	12	0	0
01-2004	12-2004	238	6	0	1
01-2005	12-2005	299	0	0	3
01-2006	12-2006	284	0	4	5
01-2007	12-2007	260	1	8	0
01-2008	12-2008	225	0	11	2
01-2009	12-2009	280	0	8	0
01-2010	12-2010	358	0	22	0
01-2011	12-2011	413	0	24	0
01-2012	12-2012	425	0	23	2
01-2013	12-2013	429	0	18	2
01-2014	12-2014	312	0	6	3
01-2015	12-2015	317	0	6	2
01-2016	12-2016	228	0	11	3
01-2017	12-2017	109	0	0	0
01-2018	12-2018	196	0	0	0
Total		**4550**	**19 (0.4%)**	**144 (3.1)**	**20 (0.43%)**

Table 1.
Showing our OPCAB results.

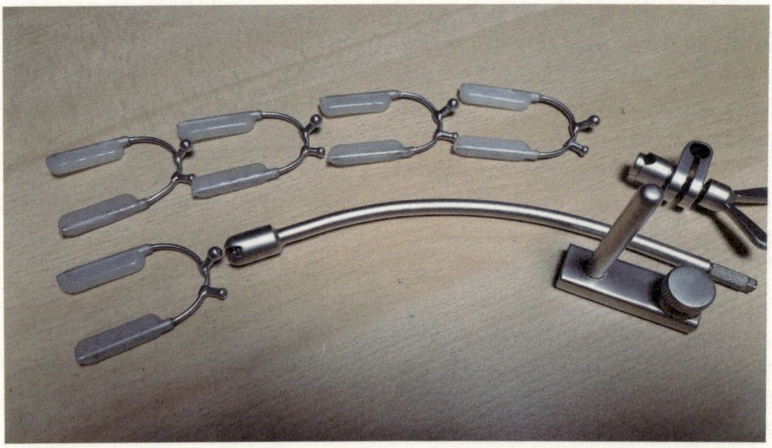

Figure 16.
Shows stabilizer with pods.

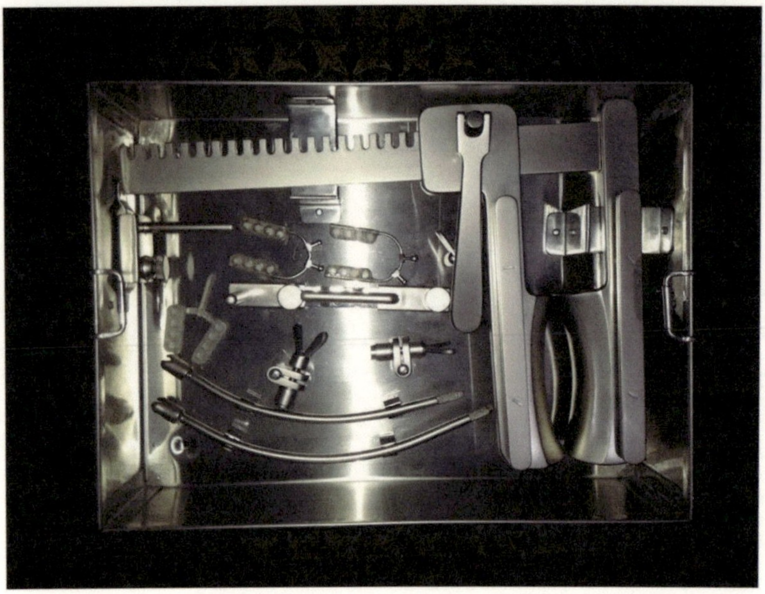

Figure 17.
Shows combo device, which comes in a box.

5.4 Simple indigenous metallic stabilizer (SIMS)

We have been using our own simple indigenous (Indian made) metallic stabilizer (SIMS) for the last 5 years or so (**Figure 16**, stabilizer and pods). It was innovated to avoid the conventional disposable plastic stabilizer that had to be changed either after every case or like in India, to change it after 10 or 20 cases. Hence we developed our own reusable, re-sterilisable metallic stabilizer, which we have used for the last 5 years even without changing the main part. The only part that has to be changed is the Pods. The pods would cost about 10–15 dollars for one pod. This has in fact reduced our carbon footprint which we leave when we do cardiac surgery [9].

The link of videos showing the SIMS in action: https://www.youtube.com/playlist?list=PLmvb6npEfabinhlatq8IYLBz8WlHo8bu1.

The SIMS comes as a combo device (**Figure 17**, shows the box, which comes with the sternal spreader and the stabilizer and its parts), which is made of a sternal spreader with a railing on both sides over which a vertical 2 inch metallic rod could be fixed with a screw and its position could be moved according to the position of the coronary artery which needed to be bypassed. Over this metal rod, we have the stabilizer rod that is fixed at its base with another clamp, which in turn could be moved over the metal rod to which ever position we need. The stabilizer rod is in fact a curved hollow metallic tube which houses another curved metal rod inside. The curved outer tube has a distal metal end that holds a housing in which the pod head could be moved around. This housing has three slots which allows the pod to move in them until it is positioned. The proximal end of the outer tube has a screw which when screwed, would tighten the inner rod. The inner rod at its distal end is convex and this moves on the concave end of the interlocking rod in front of it. The interlocking rod is the crux of the stabilizer (sent for patenting). This is a half a centimetre piece of metal which is concave on both ends. The proximal concave end allows the metal rod to push it forward or distally, and the distal concave bit allows the head of the pod to rest on it. Hence when the pod is placed parallel to the coronary artery, we first tighten the rod in the intended position and the pod is positioned by tightening the screw at the proximal end. This screw in turn pushes the inner rod forward, which in turn pushes the interlocking rod which tighten and stabilizes the head of the pod in the desired position. This, once positioned is so stable that it does not move at all. The pod has suckers like in the conventional stabilizers, which could be attached to the suction apparatus and can be used as suction stabilizer as well. Over time, once we get used to the stabilizer we can avoid the suction unless it is absolutely needed, like in positioning for right coronary artery grafting.

6. Conclusion

Revascularisation strategy is the most important part of planning for CABG. Whether it is done on the heart lung machine, or it is performed without the use of heart lung machine, it is important to first deliver a patent anastomosis. Just because some surgeons are able to do a good job, does not mean that everyone can do it. Hence one has to tailor make his own strategy of coronary revascularisation. Only by performing more and more such procedure, can we become confident on that technique. Just because the studies tell that arterial grafts have a better long term patency, and if we by performing this surgery on a patient are not able to provide a safe surgery, we should not do it. No wonder only 5% of surgeons perform total arterial grafting, and that only a handful of surgeons perform them on all patients. Likewise, just because we have been performing OPCAB in 100% of our patients over the last 12 years and that we have had no conversions on to the pump, does not mean that it is possible for all surgeons to do it [10]. Unless they have a mind-set and work hard for it to happen and that the team has been geared to perform without much issues, OPCAB would not be possible. It is important to watch such a team perform, by staying with them for at least a few weeks to learn this technique. Once the OPCAB technique is mastered, we could then strategize on what conduits to use and what permutations and combinations of conduits could be used. If we are able to perform a good OPCAB procedure then there is no need to use inotropes post operatively and that the hospital stay itself gets shortened. We have totally avoided inotropes in any patient who has undergone OPCAB in out centre, over the last 15 years.

Author details

Murali P. Vettath*, Kannan A. Vellachamy, Nitin Ganagadharan, Madhu Ravisankar, Smera Koroth and Gopalakrishnan Raman
Department of CVTS, Meitra Hospital, Kozhikode, Kerala, India

*Address all correspondence to: murali.vettath@gmail.com

References

[1] Vettath MP. Re-engineering in OPCAB—A Vettath's perspective. World Journal of Cardio vascular Disease. 2013;**2013**(3):33-44. DOI: 10.4236/wjcd.2013.34A006

[2] Takanashi S, Fukui T, Hosoda Y, Shimizu Y. Off-pump long onlay bypass grafting using left internal mammary artery for diffusely diseased coronary artery. The Annals of Thoracic Surgery. 2003;**76**:635-637

[3] Vettath MP. Vettath's anastomotic obturator: A simple proximal anastomotic device. The Heart Surgery Forum. 2003;**6**(5):366-368. Available from: www.hsforum.com/vol6/issue5/2003-73305.html

[4] Vettath MP, Kannan AV, Sheen Peecheeyen CS, Baburajan AK, Vahab A, Sujith MP. Vettath's anastomotic obturator—Our experience of 269 proximal anastamosis. Heart, Lung & Circulation. 2004;**13**:288-290

[5] Vettath MP, Ismail EK, Kannan AV. Extended use of Vettath's anastomotic obturator (vao). Surgical Science. 2011;**2**:451-452. Available from: http:www.scirp.org/journal/ss

[6] Prabhu AD, Thazhkuni IE, Rajendran S, Thamaran RA, Vellachamy KA, Vettath MP. Mammary patch reconstruction of left anterior descending coronary artery. Asian Cardiovascular & Thoracic Annals. 2008a;**16**:313-317

[7] Prabhu AD, Karim RA, Rajendran S, Thazhkuni IE, Thamaran RA, Vellachami KA, et al. Vettath's technique of long mammary patch reconstruction of a diffusely diseased left anterior descending coronary artery without endarterectomy on the beating heart. The Heart Surgery Forum. 2008;**11**(2):64-67. DOI: 10.1532/HSF98.20071155. Available from: http://cardenjennings.metapress.com

[8] Vettath M et al. Role of intra aortic balloon pump in off pump coronary artery bypass—A Vettath modification. World journal of cardiovascular disease. 2016;**6**:188-195. DOI: 10.4236/wjcd.2016.66020. Available from: http://www.scirp.org/journal/wjcd

[9] Vettath MP, Kannan AV, Nitin G, Ravisankar M, Smera K, Gopalakrishnan R. Development of SIMS (simple indigenous metallic stabilizer) for OPCAB. World Journal of Cardiovascular Diseases. 2019;**9**: 324-330. DOI: 10.4236/wjcd.201. ISSN Online: 2164-5337 ISSN. Available from: http://www.scirp.org/journal/wjcd

[10] Vettath MP, Ravisankar M, Kopjar T, Kannan AV, Gangadharan N. Off-pump coronary artery bypass grafting improves early clinical outcomes including operative mortality. The Heart Surgery Forum. 2018;**21**(3):E151-E157. DOI: 10.1532/hsf.2007

Chapter 8

Surgical Treatment of Hypertrophic Obstructive Cardiomyopathy

Francesca Nicolo', Antonio Lio, Marina Comisso, Romina Pantanella, Roberto Scrofani and Francesco Musumeci

Abstract

Hypertrophic cardiomyopathy is a genetic disorder of the myocardium, characterized by marked myocardial hypertrophy that may lead to the development of symptoms such as dyspnea, angina pectoris, or stress-induced syncopes, with an increased risk of sudden cardiac death, due to obstruction of the left ventricular outflow tract (hypertrophic obstructive cardiomyopathy). Septal reduction treatment is needed in these patients, in order to relieve of the symptoms. In addition, mitral valve apparatus should be assessed in these patients, in order to recognize a dynamic movement of the MV during systole anteriorly toward the LVOT. In this chapter, we will describe the current surgical management of HOCM.

Keywords: hypertrophic obstructive cardiomyopathy, HOCM, myotomy, SAM

1. Introduction

Hypertrophic cardiomyopathy (HCM) is a genetic disorder of the myocardium, characterized by marked myocardial hypertrophy (>15 mm) that cannot be explained by any other diseases that may cause secondary hypertrophy [1]. Its prevalence is 0.2–0.6% [2], with an overall annual mortality rate of 1%.

People with HCM often remain oligosymptomatic or even asymptomatic for many years; anyway, they may develop as cardinal symptoms dyspnea, angina pectoris, or stress-induced syncopes, with an increased risk of sudden cardiac death, particularly in young people and athletes [3], due to obstruction of the left ventricular outflow tract (LVOT). This obstruction is dynamic and largely influenced by changes in left ventricular loading and contractility, with subsequently increased left ventricular systolic pressure and secondary mitral regurgitation (MR), myocardial ischemia, and reduction in cardiac output. Around 70% of patients with HCM display relevant obstruction (HOCM) with a high peak pressure difference (more than 30 mm Hg) [4]; in half of these patients the obstruction is present even at rest, while in the remainder it is latent, so that a gradient can be demonstrated only under stress. Septal reduction treatments can lead to considerable relief of the symptoms even in patients whose obstruction is latent.

Echocardiography is an important and reliable method for diagnosing HOCM and for planning the kind of treatment. Echocardiography enables determination of the extent of the left ventricular hypertrophy and of the site, severity, and

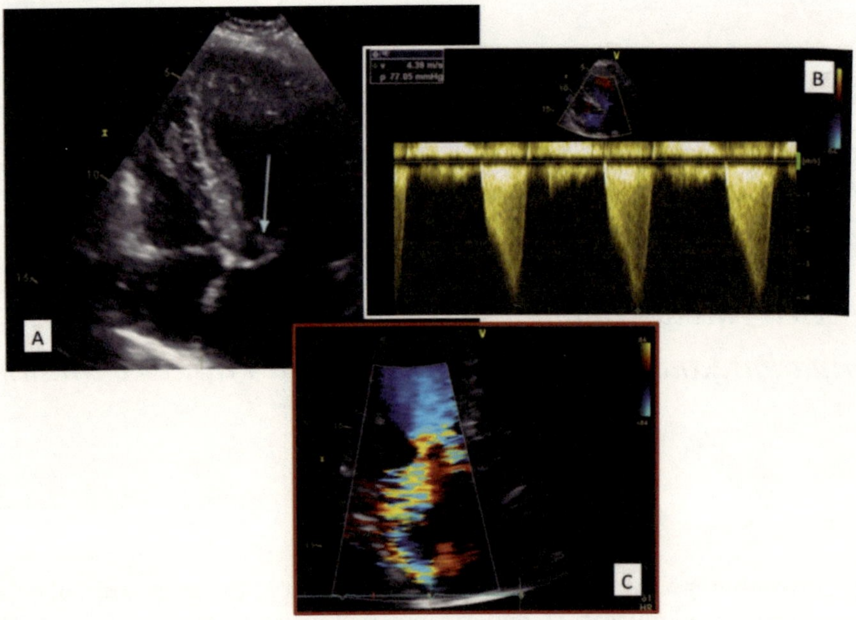

Figure 1.
Transthoracic echocardiography showing LVOT obstruction (A), with a resting LVOT gradient of 77 mmHg (B) and severe MR, due to SAM (C). Figure courtesy of non-invasive cardiology diagnostic laboratory, Cardiology Department, L. Sacco Hospital, Via G.B. Grassi 74, Milano, Italy.

mechanism of any obstruction. In addition, mitral valve (MV) apparatus can be adequately studied, in order to recognize any systolic distortion of the MV associated with systolic anterior motion (SAM) that often leads to secondary MR (**Figure 1**).

Despite medical therapy (treatment with B-blockers or, sometimes, Verapamil) is the first-line therapy for symptomatic patients with LVOT obstruction [1], a large proportion of patients with dynamic obstruction remain symptomatic so, a septal reduction treatment (SRT) is needed in order to relief of the symptoms. This can take the form of either septal myectomy or percutaneous alcohol ablation of the septum [5]. In this chapter we will describe the current surgical management of HOCM.

2. Anatomical classification of HCM

Morphology is variable, common variants being basal, mid-ventricular, apical, and diffuse types have been described. Maron classification reported 4 variants of HCM [6]:

- Type 1: hypertrophy (10% of patients) confined to the anterior portion of the ventricular septum;

- Type 2: hypertrophy (20% of patients), involves the anterior and posterior portion of the ventricular septum;

- Type 3: hypertrophy (52% of patients), involves the anterior and posterior portion of the ventricular septum as well as the lateral free wall;

- Type 4: hypertrophy (18% of patients), involves left ventricular regions other than the anterior septum and the posterior free wall.

3. Surgical indication

ACC/AHA and ESC guidelines recommend that septal reduction therapy should be performed only by experienced operators, working as part of a multidisciplinary team expert, in the management of HCM [1, 7]. A SRT should be performed in presence of:

1. Significant LVOT obstruction (resting or maximum provoked LVOT gradient of ≥50 mmHg)

2. Angina, Dyspnea (NYHA functional class III-IV), Syncope

3. Persistent symptoms on maximal medical therapy.

4. The current indications have expanded recently to include symptomatic patients with low resting outflow gradients and latent obstruction.

4. Surgical approaches

1. Standard median sternotomy

2. Ministernotomy

3. Right anterolateral minithoracotomy (IV I.S.)

5. Surgical septal myectomy

Surgical septal myectomy is the therapeutic gold standard for the treatment of drug-refractory disabling symptoms in HCM caused by LVOT obstruction. This procedure can relieve hemodynamic disorders and has an acceptable surgical risk when performed on appropriate patients and in experienced centers [7].

It was performed, for the first time, in 1968 by Morrow et al. [8]; initially, the myectomy was limited in scope, but nowadays the resection is much more aggressive in terms of both width and length [5, 9]. Sparing the cardiac conduction system, septal myocardium is resected, depending on the area of hypertrophy and extending if necessary as far as the level of the papillary muscles, to an extent sufficient to eliminate the obstruction, retaining septal thickness of 1 cm. Surgical septal myectomy can be performed as follows:

5.1 Transaortic extended septal myectomy (TAESM)

TAESM through a transverse aortotomy, the aortic valve is totally exposed and the aortic leaflets are retracted so as to inspect the LVOT, the hypertrophic cardiac muscle and anterior MV leaflet. In order to open the LVOT and reduce the gradient to <30 mmHg, resection of the hypertrophic muscle until the thickness of the LV wall and interventricular septum became nearly normal by visual inspection, has to be performed. The myectomy should be initiated about 1.5 cm below the aortic annulus starting at the level of the non-coronary/right-coronary commissure to avoid the membranous septum and avoid creating a secondary ventricular septal defect (VSD). The septum is cut into as much as possible to relieve the obstruction and it is extended toward the left/non-coronary commissure so that the entire

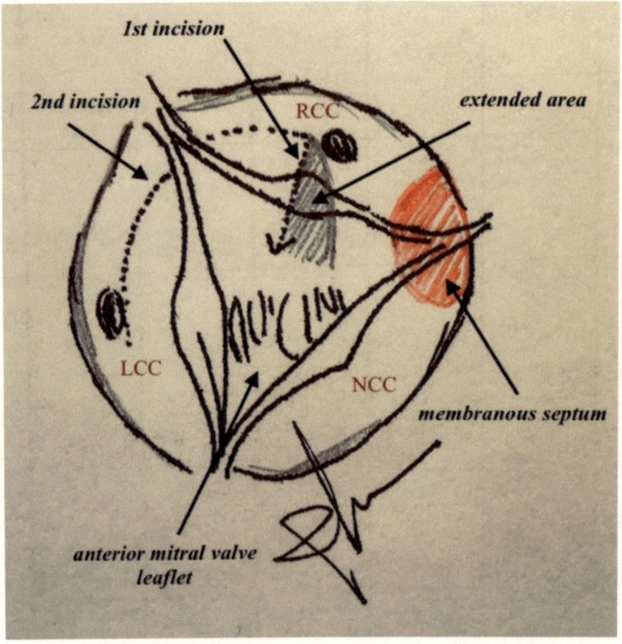

Figure 2.
Extension of the resection under the membranous septum.

septum is trimmed off all around (**Figure 2**). The TAESM is the most commonly used technique and it has been associated with very low mortality, consistent alleviation of outflow gradients and excellent long-term survival [10].

5.2 Transmitral septal myectomy (TMSM)

The MV is approached through the left atrium, in the interatrial groove. Then, the base of the AL is widely detached from commissure to commissure, with the septum that lies just in front of the surgeon. The myectomy is continued further toward the apex with at least 1 cm depth of muscle removed. The anterior MV leaflet is then reconstructed (sometimes using an autologous pericardial patch with the size of the patch that should be as biggest as possible, in order to move posteriorly toward the left ventricle the coaptation plane). This approach is useful for those patients with diffuse hypertrophy extending to or below the papillary muscles with midcavity muscular obstruction: these patients are suboptimal candidates for the Morrow procedure. Benefits of the transmitral exposure include a wide view of the ventricular septum, absent risk of injury to the aortic valve cusps, and the opportunity to address concomitant abnormalities of the MV and subvalvular apparatus.

5.3 Complete septal myectomy by a double approach (aortic and mitral)

In patients with simultaneous MR due to SAM, the insufficiency is almost always reduced or eliminated by myectomy alone. Sometimes, there may be associated a lesion of the aortic valve and/or fibrous subaortic stenosis; these also require surgical correction, depending on their severity. Intraoperative echocardiography helps the surgeon to determine the individual extent of the disease and decide on the necessary scope of resection.

More difficult to treat are patients with an apical variant of HCM; they have obliteration of the left ventricular chamber with severe diastolic dysfunction. The results of myectomy depend essentially on the experience and competence of the surgeon. Only in specialized centers can myectomy be carried out with a risk of perioperative complications under 1%. The hemodynamic results are usually excellent with a postoperative gradient <10 mm Hg [11]. VSD, atrioventricular block and residual obstruction may complicate a septal myotomy; anyway, incidence is lower for experienced surgeons with a risk <3% in expert hands [12]. Long-term results following surgery are good, with more than 90% of patients being asymptomatic [13]. Septal myectomy is the gold standard in SRT, because of fewer complications and better freedom from redo procedures, with a better long term outcome rather than septal ablation.

6. Adjuncts to septal myectomy

6.1 SAM correction

SAM describes the dynamic movement of the MV during systole anteriorly toward the LVOT. It occurs in 31–61% of HCM patients, and it is associated with resting LVOT obstruction in 25–50% of them [14].

SAM-mediated MR typically resolves with extended myectomy alone, anyway, a well comprehension of all the mechanisms that can predispose to or precipitate SAM, is important, in order to treat this mechanism. Factors predisposing to SAM are:

a. structural anomalies such as:

- small left ventricular chamber
- bulging septum
- chordal anomaly
- papillary muscle displacement
- redundant anterior or posterior leaflets

b. geometric factors such as:

- annular undersizing
- anterior displacement of MV (any anatomical or surgical translocation of the MV anteriorly will increase the forces acting to draw the MV anteriorly that may precipitate SAM)
- low anterior—posterior (A-P) length ratio (A-P leaflet length ratio <1.3 is a risk factor for SAM)
- reduced mitral-aortic angle (<15°)
- distance reduction between MV coaptation point and septum

c. kinetic factors such as

- hyperdynamic left ventricle (LV)

Surgical techniques proposed to correct concomitant SAM in HOCM are:

- *Changes to posterior leaflet height*, in order to avoid anterior shifting of the coaptation point closer to the base of the anterior leaflet, which predispose to SAM [15]. The resulting posterior mitral leaflet (PML) should have a reduced height of 1 cm:

    - o triangular resection of PML and ventricularization [16];

    - o sliding posterior leaflet plasty technique (moves the coaptation point posteriorly) [17] (**Figures 3–5**);

    - o modified sliding leaflet technique (middle scallop of PML is resected, differs from Carpentier in eliminating triangular resection) [18] (**Figure 6**);

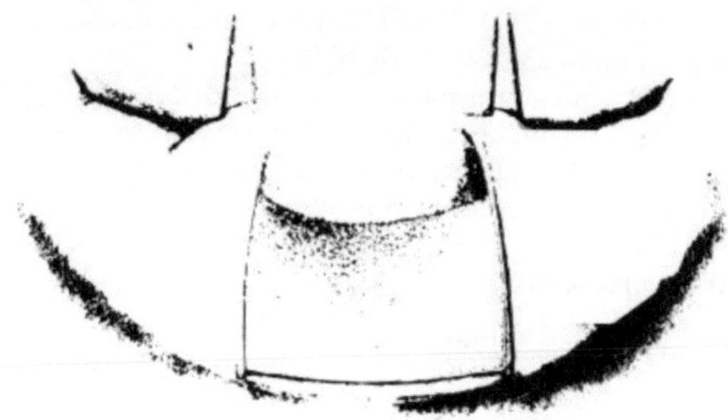

Figure 3.
Quadrangular P2 resection. Adapted from the book "Reconstructive Valve Surgery", by Carpentier et al. 2010, Imprint: Saunders, Copyright: © Saunders 2010.

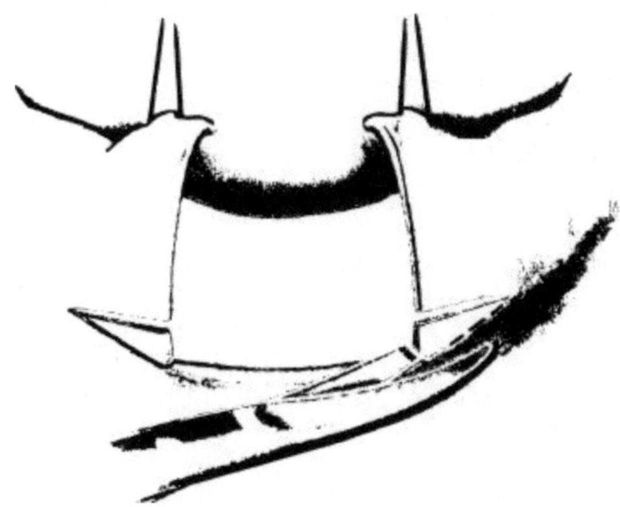

Figure 4.
Quadrangular P2 resection + sliding plasty. Adapted from the book "Reconstructive Valve Surgery", by Carpentier et al. 2010, Imprint: Saunders, Copyright: © Saunders 2010.

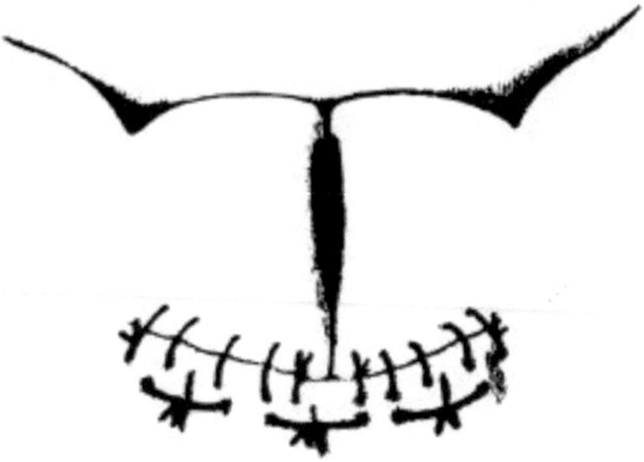

Figure 5.
Final result of quadrangular P2 resection + sliding plasty. Adapted from the book "Reconstructive Valve Surgery", by Carpentier et al. 2010, Imprint: Saunders, Copyright: © Saunders 2010.

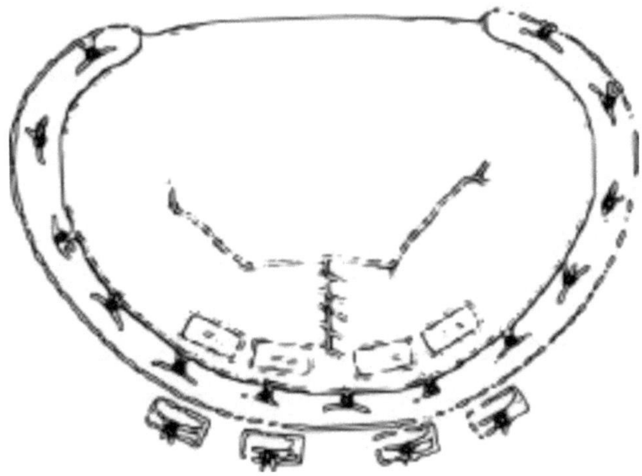

Figure 6.
Posterior mitral valve leaflet shortening.

- PML folding plasty [19];
- Loop technique (height adjustment of the mitral leaflets using artificial chordae: after artificial chordae and annuloplasty ring placement in the normal way, a polyester reduction suture with a spaghetti loop supporting it is placed on the posterior leaflet surface, and tied down until its height is <1.5 cm), [20] (**Figure 7**);
- chordal translocation (PML secondary chordae are transected and moved to the AML) [21];
- edge-to-edge, or Alfieri stitch technique (A1-P1 stitch instead of midline) [22].

- *Changes to anterior leaflet height*, in order to reduce the redundant leaflet and, subsequently, the A-P length ratio (risk factor for SAM development):

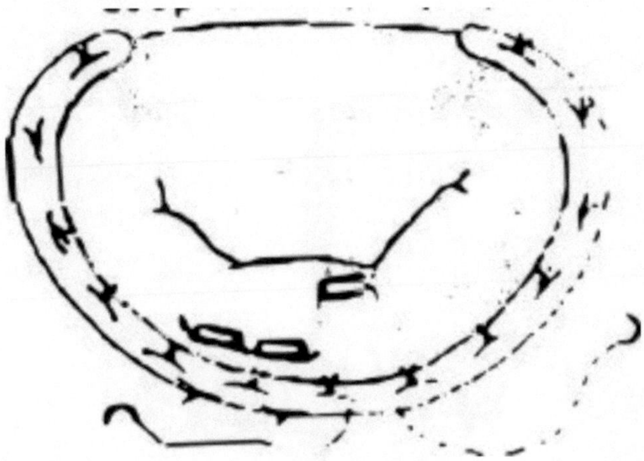

Figure 7.
Loop technique.

- ◦ elliptical excision of the anterior mitral leaflet (excision site is then closed with double-layer prolene stitches) [23];
- ◦ elliptical excision with repositioning of major basal chords [24];
- ◦ removal of accessory chordae that may tether the AML to the septum, resulting in SAM [25].

- *Annuloplasty ring sizes*: any reduction in annular circumference reduces the mitral—aortic angle, which increases the risk of SAM, so an annular undersizing should not be performed, in order to maintain the coaptation plane as much as possible away from the septum:
    - ◦ annular enlargement (post-MV repair, especially in Barlow's disease): 36–40 mm annular rings are used in presence of excessive mitral tissue [26];
    - ◦ annular plication: plication sutures are used to tie down the PML to the annulus [27];
- "*Resection-plication-release*": in HCM, the concomitant use of myectomy, plication of the AML and release of the papillary muscles remodels the LV in order to reduce SAM [28].
- *Mitral valve replacement*: if SAM is severe and persistent despite exhaustive medical and surgical attempts at eliminating SAM, MV replacement can be the only option. In this setting, care must be taken to properly resect any remaining mitral tissue, to prevent SAM recurring.

6.2 Arrhythmia surgery

Patients with HCM are at increased risk of development of atrial fibrillation due to long-standing elevation of the left ventricular end-diastolic and left atrial pressures with subsequent left atrial chamber enlargement. Anyway, there is little evidence to support the addition of the Cox-maze procedure to septal myectomy.

6.3 Management of papillary muscle abnormalities

Sometimes, LVOT obstruction is present after septal myectomy because of anomalies of the (MV) valve apparatus: an accessory papillary muscle that arises from the ventricular septum and that is attached to the side of the anterior leaflet, may be present. In these patients, the accessory muscle has to be excised in its entirety. Other anomalies of the mitral apparatus may be the presence of accessory papillary muscles, or fusion of the anterior papillary muscle with the ventricular septum or left-ventricular free wall, or the presence of abnormal chordae tendineae that attach to the ventricular septum or to the free wall; all of this abnormalities may contribute to a persistent LVOT gradient and should be corrected in order to perform an adequate SRT.

In HCM, the anterior and inward displacement of papillary muscles is thought to create diastolic downwards vortex forces which pull the MV into the LVOT [29].

6.4 Management of concomitant MV disease

Degenerative MV disease requires attention at the time of myectomy in contrast to SAM-mediated MR that typically resolves with extended myectomy alone.

In our experience, when a concomitant mitral valve repair (MVR) is needed, we use a flexible posterior band that is slightly upsized, in order to minimize or avoid potential development of SAM postoperatively.

7. Other indications for septal myectomy

Apical and midventricular variants of HCM are difficult entities to diagnose and treat medically, with the only alternative to myectomy being heart transplantation.

8. Septal myectomy versus alcohol septal ablation

Despite an extended surgical septal myectomy is considered the gold standard for managing symptomatic patients [1], percutaneous alcohol ablation of the septum has emerged as an alternative to surgical septal myectomy [30]. In this approach, alcohol is injected into the first septal perforator in order to create a localized myocardial infarction. The advantages of this non surgical procedures are a faster recovery with a subsequent quick return to daily lifestyle; anyway, the literature tends to support better long-term symptom relief in those patients who undergo septal myectomy [31] with a higher procedural success and a lower rate of complications when myectomy is performed in experienced centers compared with alcohol septal ablation. In addition, we have to keep in mind that young patients and patients with severe or relatively thin septal thickness and a very high LVOT gradient are considered poor candidates for the percutaneous approach. Importantly, surgical septal myectomy also facilitates the correction of other abnormalities of the LVOT and repair of associated abnormalities of the MV and anomalous papillary muscles that can also contribute to residual dynamic outflow tract obstruction.

9. Conclusions

Due to the complex ventricular phenotype of septal hypertrophy which increases the drag forces acting on the MV, and also due to primary MV anomalies, a multifaceted approach to repair and abolition of LVOT obstruction is required in HOCM. Septal myectomy is fundamental and represent the first step to any of these. In addition, specific techniques for SAM in the context of HOCM have been described. Each technique proposed for the surgical correction of HOCM has evolved to meet a specific anatomical problem, so it is inappropriate to rate one surgical procedure as superior to another; anyway, repair which resects as little tissue as possible and that does not distort the anatomy significantly should be preferred. Surgeons must understand the anatomical cause of LVOT obstruction, and this should guide them to the choice of the technique to adopt. Ease of repair should be also considered, as this will have beneficial consequences for the total time under cardiopulmonary bypass.

Alcohol septal ablation for HCM has been proposed as a less-invasive alternative to surgical myectomy, although its role in the management of HCM associated with SAM requires further investigations so that, the current evidence, supports the use of septal myectomy in the clinical practice [32].

Acknowledgements

The authors would like to thank Francesco Ballarin, Ph.D., assistant professor in Numerical Analysis, SISSA mathLab, International School for Advanced Studies, Trieste, Italy, for imaging elaboration.

Conflict of interest

None.

Author details

Francesca Nicolo'[1*], Antonio Lio[1], Marina Comisso[1], Romina Pantanella[2], Roberto Scrofani[3] and Francesco Musumeci[1]

1 Department of Cardiac Surgery and Transplantation, S. Camillo Hospital, Rome, Italy

2 Department of Cardiac Surgery, Policlinico Sant'Andrea, Sapienza University, Rome, Italy

3 Department of Cardiac Surgery, L. Sacco Hospital, Milano, Italy

*Address all correspondence to: nicolo_francy84@hotmail.it

References

[1] Authors/Task Force Members, Elliott PM, Anastasakis A, et al. 2014 ESC guidelines on diagnosis and management of hypertrophic cardiomyopathy: The task force for the diagnosis and management of hypertrophic cardiomyopathy of the European Society of Cardiology (ESC). European Heart Journal. 2014;**35**:2733-2779

[2] Semsarian C, Ingles J, Maron MS, Maron BJ. New perspectives on the prevalence of hypertrophic cardiomyopathy. Journal of the American College of Cardiology. 2015;**65**:1249-1254

[3] Maron BJ. Sudden death in hypertrophic cardiomyopathy. Journal of Cardiovascular Translational Research. 2009;**2**:368-380

[4] Prinz C, Farr M, Hering D, Horstkotte D, Faber L. The diagnosis and treatment of hypertrophic cardiomyopathy. Deutsches Ärzteblatt International. 2011;**108**:209-215

[5] Nishimura RA, Seggewiss H, Schaff HV. Hypertrophic obstructive cardiomyopathy: Surgical myectomy and septal ablation. Circulation Research. 2017;**121**:771-783

[6] Maron BJ, Gottdiener JS, Epstein SE. Patterns and significance of distribution of left ventricular hypertrophy in hypertrophic cardiomyopathy. A wide angle, two dimensional echocardiographic study of 125 patients. The American Journal of Cardiology. 1981;**48**:418-428

[7] Gersh BJ, Maron BJ, Bonow RO, et al. 2011 CCF/AHA guideline for the diagnosis and treatment of hypertrophic cardiomyopathy: Executive summary: A report of the American college of cardiology foundation/American heart association task force on practice guidelines. The Journal of Thoracic and Cardiovascular Surgery. 2011;**142**:1303-1338

[8] Morrow AG, Brockenbrough EC. Surgical treatment of idiopathic hypertrophic subaortic stenosis: Technic and hemodynamic results of subaortic ventriculomyotomy. Annals of Surgery. 1961;**154**:181-189

[9] Messmer BJ. Extended myectomy for hypertrophic obstructive cardiomyopathy. The Annals of Thoracic Surgery. 1994;**58**:575-577

[10] Smedira NG, Lytle BW, Lever HM, Rajeswaran J, Krishnaswamy G, Kaple RK, et al. Current effectiveness and risks of isolated septal myectomy for hypertrophic obstructive cardiomyopathy. The Annals of Thoracic Surgery. 2008;**85**:127-133

[11] Maron BJ, Dearani JA, Ommen SR, et al. Low operative mortality achieved with surgical septal myectomy: Role of dedicated hypertrophic cardiomyopathy centers in the management of dynamic subaortic obstruction. Journal of the American College of Cardiology. 2015;**66**:1307-1308

[12] Kim LK, Swaminathan RV, Looser P, et al. Hospital volume outcomes after septal myectomy and alcohol septal ablation for treatment of obstructive hypertrophic cardiomyopathy: US nationwide inpatient database, 2003-2011. JAMA Cardiology. 2016;**1**:324-332

[13] Mohr R, Schaff HV, Puga FJ, Danielson GK. Results of operation for hypertrophic obstructive cardiomyopathy in children and adults less than 40 years of age. Circulation. 1989;**80**:I191-I196

[14] Maron BJ, Peterson EE, Maron MS, Peterson JE. Prevalence of hypertrophic cardiomyopathy in an

outpatient population referred for echocardiographic study. The American Journal of Cardiology. 1994;**73**:577-580

[15] Carpentier A. The sliding leaflet technique. Le Club Mitral Newsletter. 1998;**4**:1-5

[16] Suri RM, Burkhart HM, Schaff HV. A novel method of leaflet reconstruction after triangular resection for posterior mitral valve prolapse. The Annals of Thoracic Surgery. 2010;**89**:e53-e56

[17] Jebara VA, Mihaileanu S, Acar C, Brizard C, Grare P, Latremouille C, et al. Left ventricular outflow tract obstruction after mitral valve repair. Results of the sliding leaflet technique. Circulation. 1993;**88**:II30-II34

[18] Gillinov AM, Cosgrove DM III. Modified sliding leaflet technique for repair of the mitral valve. The Annals of Thoracic Surgery. 1999;**68**:2356-2357

[19] Grossi EA, Galloway AC, Kallenbach K, Miller JS, Esposito R, Schwartz DS, et al. Early results of posterior leaflet folding plasty for mitral valve reconstruction. The Annals of Thoracic Surgery. 1998;**65**:1057-1059

[20] Kudo M, Yozu R, Kokaji K, Kimura N. A simple method of prevention for systolic anterior motion in mitral valve repair by loop technique method. The Annals of Thoracic Surgery. 2009;**87**:324-325

[21] Sternik L, Zehr KJ. Systolic anterior motion of the mitral valve after mitral valve repair: A method of prevention. Texas Heart Institute Journal. 2005;**32**:47-49

[22] Gillinov AM, Smedira NG, Shiota T. Use of the Alfieri edge-to-edge technique to eliminate left ventricular outflow tract obstruction caused by mitral systolic anterior motion. The Annals of Thoracic Surgery. 2004;**78**:e92-e93

[23] Shah PM, Raney AA. Echocardiographic correlates of left ventricular outflow obstruction and systolic anterior motion following mitral valve repair. The Journal of Heart Valve Disease. 2001;**10**:302-306

[24] Raney AA, Shah PM, Joyo CI. The 'Pomeroy procedure': A new method to correct post-mitral valve repair systolic anterior motion. The Journal of Heart Valve Disease. 2001;**10**:307-311

[25] Massaccesi S, Mancinelli G, Munch C, Catania S, Iacobone G, Piccoli GP. Functional systolic anterior motion of the mitral valve due to accessory chordae. Journal of Cardiovascular Medicine (Hagerstown, Md.). 2008;**9**:105-108

[26] Adams DH, Anyanwu AC, Rahmanian PB, Abascal V, Salzberg SP, Filsoufi F. Large annuloplasty rings facilitate mitral valve repair in Barlow's disease. The Annals of Thoracic Surgery. 2006;**82**:2096-2100

[27] Mesana T, Ibrahim M, Hynes M. A technique for annular plication to facilitate sliding plasty after extensive mitral valve posterior leaflet resection. The Annals of Thoracic Surgery. 2005;**79**:720-722

[28] Balaram SK, Tyrie L, Sherrid MV, Afthinos J, Hillel Z, Winson G, et al. Resection—plication—release for hypertrophic cardiomyopathy: Clinical and echocardiographic follow-up. The Annals of Thoracic Surgery. 2008;**86**:1539-1544

[29] Lefebvre XP, He S, Levine RA, Yoganathan AP. Systolic anterior motion of the mitral valve in hypertrophic cardiomyopathy: An in vitro pulsatile flow study. The Journal of Heart Valve Disease. 1995;**4**:422-438

[30] Goel K, Schaff HV, Nishimura RA. Natural history of apical hyper trophic cardiomyopathy and novel surgical treatment. The Journal of Thoracic and Cardiovascular Surgery. 2016;**152**:626-627

[31] Marian AJ, Braunwald E. Hypertrophic cardiomyopathy: Genetics, pathogenesis, clinical manifestations, diagnosis, and therapy. Circulation Research. 2017;**121**:749-770

[32] Alam M, Dokainish H, Lakkis N. Alcohol septal ablation for hypertrophic obstructive cardiomyopathy: A systematic review of published studies. Journal of Interventional Cardiology. 2006;**19**:319-327

Chapter 9

Transcatheter Cardiac Surgery

Antonio Giovanni Cammardella, Federico Ranocchi, Antonio Lio, Amedeo Pergolini, Francesco Nicolò, Marina Comisso, Vitaliano Buffa and Francesco Musumeci

Abstract

The introduction of transcatheter aortic valve implantation (TAVI) have changed the management of patients affected by severe aortic stenosis. Nowadays, TAVI procedure represents the treatment of choice in patients with severe AS inoperable or at high risk. MDCT is the technique of choice in preoperative planning: it provides information regarding aortic valve and vascular access. Particular attention should be paid on bicuspid valve morphology. The choice of valve is, basically, based on confidence and experience of the operator and center.

Keywords: transcatheter aortic valve implantation, aortic stenosis, patient selection, imaging, access site

1. Introduction

The introduction of transcatheter aortic valve implantation (TAVI) has changed the management of patients affected by severe aortic stenosis.

The calculated incidence rate of severe AS is 4.4‰/year in patients ≥65 years [1]. The prevalence of the disease was estimated of about 13% in general population aged ≥75 years [2].

Approximately 40% of symptomatic severe AS patients do not undergo SAVR [1].

Nowadays, TAVI procedure represents the treatment of choice in patients with severe AS inoperable or at high risk. The improvement in early and midterm results has extended the indication for TAVI also to elderly patients at intermediate and low risk for surgery. This is the result of a continuous improvement in patients' selection and procedural assessment which is supported by the progress in imaging technology which is central for better diagnostic planning and more precise technical procedure.

2. Selection of patients

Actually, the main surgical risk score used in clinical practice and in randomized trial is the STS score: a STS score > 8% identifies patient at high risk; a STS score between 4 and 8% corresponds to an intermediate-risk profile; a STS lower than 4% encloses patients at low surgical risk [3].

The last 2017 ESC/EACTS guidelines for the management of valvular disease recommend that in patients who are at increased surgical risk, the decision between SAVR and TAVI should be made by the Heart Team, according to the individual patient characteristics, with TAVI being favored in elderly patients suitable for transfemoral access (class of recommendation Ib) [4].

AHA/ACC guidelines, also, underline the importance of a multidisciplinary Heart Team in the evaluation of a patient affected by severe AS [5].

However, it seems to be clear that the only evaluation based on surgical preoperative risk score (STS or Euroscore II) is not enough. In fact, specific risk factors for TAVI, such as frailty, chest radiation, porcelain aorta, and vessel tortuosity are not included [6]. Thus, it is difficult to create an appropriate risk score for TAVI due to heterogeneity of patient characteristics.

In conclusion, the role of the Heart Team to include a cardiac surgeon, a cardiologist with interest in heart valve disease and an interventional cardiologist, other specialist such as anesthesiologists and geriatricians, and, if necessary, other clinicians for a complete patient assessment is fundamental [6].

3. Imaging assessment

The use of multidetector computed tomography (MDCT) is a daily practice in the preoperative planning of TAVI. MDCT improves the precision in prosthesis sizing and reduce peripheral vascular complications [3].

MDCT provides information about aortic annulus, LVOT calcifications, valve morphology, coronary ostial height, sinus of Valsalva, sino-tubular junction, ascending aorta, and optimal projection curve.

Moreover, through MDCT it is possible to have an analysis of coronary arteries status: if it detects significant coronary stenosis, a coronary angiography should be performed.

MDCT has a key role in vascular access assessment: by routine use of CT scan in preprocedural planning, the rate of vascular complication has dropped to 4–5%.

3.1 Aortic annulus

The aortic annulus is defined as the luminal contour within a virtual plane aligned with the most basal attachment points of the three aortic valve cusps [7]. Usually, the annulus can be measured into the systole, corresponding to 30–40% of the R-R interval: in this way the under-sizing of the prostheses can be avoided [3].

The measurement of the aortic annulus can be obtained manually or semiautomatically. It is clear that the support of software facilitates the work, but it requires a supervision by an expert operator.

In the manual procedure, once the central axis is aligned with the long axis of the aortic root, turning counterclockwise, the lower insertions of the single cusps are identified (**Figure 1**).

Once aortic annulus is obtained, the measurements of minimal and maximal diameter, perimeter, and area can be calculated (**Figure 2**).

Next, we can proceed to measure coronaries' height, inter-commissural distances, sino-tubular junction, and ascending aorta diameters (**Figure 2**).

It is very important to identify LVOT calcifications, their distribution, and their protrusions. The amount of calcium in LVOT is correlated with AV blocks and annular rupture, representing one of the factors keeping in mind the choice of the type of prostheses (balloon-expandable or self-expanding).

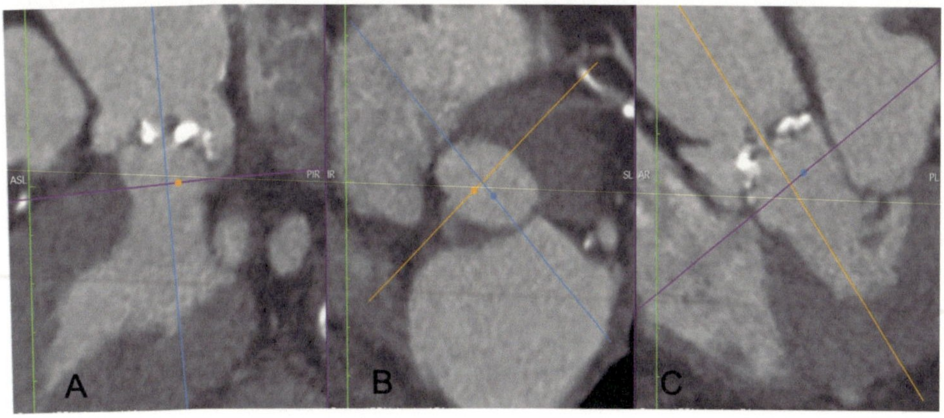

Figure 1.
Aortic annulus (virtual basal ring) in sagittal view (A), axial (B), and coronal (C).

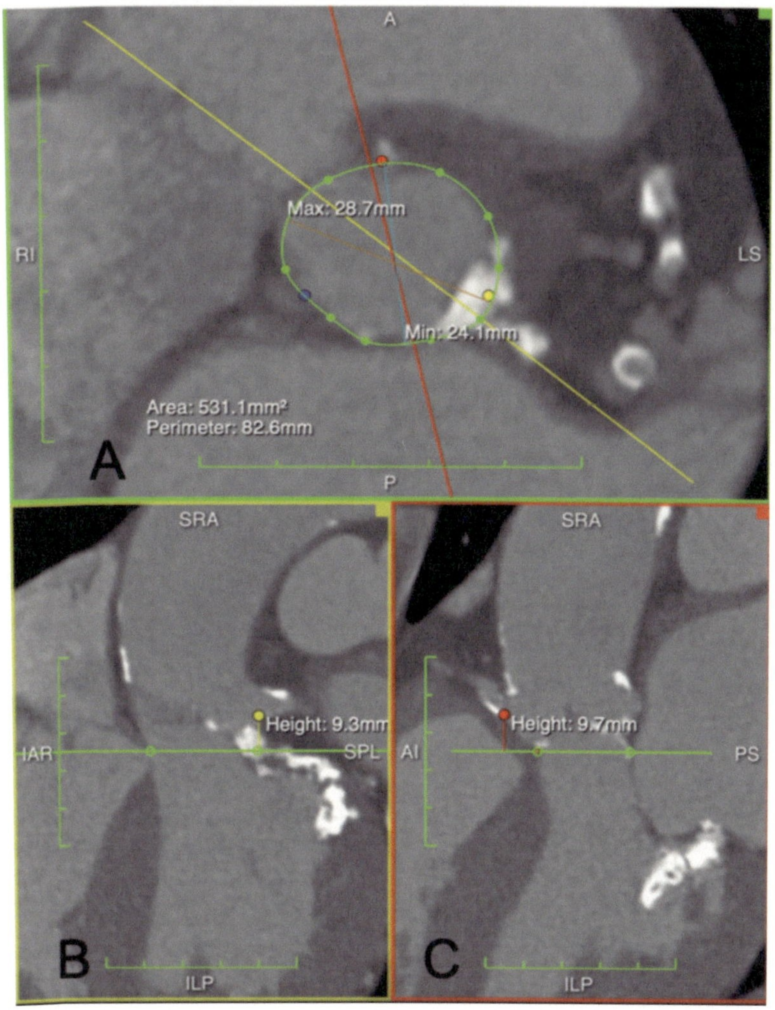

Figure 2.
(A) aortic annulus. (B) Left main height. (C) Right coronary height.

3.2 Bicuspid aortic valve

The incidence of bicuspid aortic valve (BAV) is up to 2–3% in the general population, but probably echocardiography underestimates the real percentage [8]. In the USA, Transcatheter Valve Therapy registry, 2% of the patients had BAVs [9].

According to the number of cusps, the presence of raphes, and the orientation, bicuspid aortic valve was classified into three types (0, 1, 2) and in subcategories [10]. A novel non-numerical classification seems to be useful in TAVI procedure. This classification identifies three BAV morphologies: tri-commissural (one commissure completely fused between two cusps), bi-commissural raphe type (two cusps fused by a fibrous or calcified ridge of various height), and bi-commissural non-raphe type (two cusps completely fused; there are only two commissures and no raphe or third commissure) [11].

For a long time, BAV was considered a risk condition in TAVI procedures. The association between BAV and some risk factors for TAVI is clear: calcified raphe, asymmetrical annulus, the risk of annulus rupture, coronary obstruction, and paravalvular leaks (PVL). Moreover, it is relevant to underline that BAV is associated more frequently with aortopathy (ascending aorta aneurism and coarctation). Thus, it is important to investigate these conditions prior to TAVI, because they should be a contraindication to implantation [6].

In addition, the height and location of coronary ostia in BAV could be very different than in tricuspid valves, and a specific assessment is fundamental to avoid coronary occlusion. About that, in those cases in which there is an uncertain sizing, a pre-dilatation angiography with one or more undersized balloon could be useful.

In BAV, the implantation is associated with lower success rate and higher rate of PVL, but similar outcomes, especially with new generations of prostheses [9, 12]. No significant differences were observed comparing the results of balloon-expandable to that of self-expanding valves [12].

3.3 Coronary disease

Observational data suggest that coronary artery disease (CAD) co-exists in up to 60% of patients candidate for TAVI [13]. Recent multicenter trials also report these percentages [14, 15].

Currently, the decision to perform PCI is discussed in Heart Team, considering the location and the complexity of PCI, as the latest ESC guidelines suggest.

Actually, severe lesions (>70%) involving proximal segments of coronary arteries should be treated prior to TAVI [4].

After all, it should be kept in mind that the use of FFR and iFR is theoretically influenced by the presence of a low aortic pressure due to severe aortic stenosis.

When a revascularization is required in TAVI candidates, it can be performed before TAVI, in a single procedure or after TAVI. Recent evidences showed no clinical advantages in terms of cardiovascular mortality, stroke, myocardial infarction, and acute kidney injury, when PCI is performed before or concomitant to TAVI procedure [16].

On the other hand, performing PCI after TAVI can be challenging because of the presence of valve struts and the relative difficulty to access coronary ostia. For this, the decision should be individualized on each case.

3.4 Vascular access

The choice of the most appropriate vascular access represents a key role in TAVI procedure. It is fundamental to evaluate the thoracoabdominal aorta, carotid arteries, and iliofemoral vessels.

Different vascular sites can be chosen: transfemoral (TF), transapical (TA), transaortic (TAo), trans-subclavian (TS), trans-carotid (Tc), and others [3, 17].

Different studies and registries have shown that a non-transfemoral TAVI accesses may be necessary up to 10–15% of patients. This is due, mainly, to obstructive peripheral vascular disease, severe vessel tortuosity, aortic aneurysm or atheroma, and previous peripheral grafts [18].

3.4.1 Transfemoral TAVI

The transfemoral access represents the preferred route in TAVI patients: because of its minimal invasiveness and large feasibility, TF access is recommended as first choice [18]. Analysis of iliofemoral vessel size, calcification, and tortuosity is necessary to establish if TF access can be used or not [19].

Multidetector CT provides all these aspects with a greater predictive value for vascular complications than invasive angiography [20].

The combination of a very small iliofemoral artery diameter and the presence of moderate or severe calcifications is associated with a high rate of vascular complications.

The minimum iliofemoral vessel diameter required is 5 mm for current self-expanding valves and 5.5 mm for balloon-expandable prostheses (ideally 6.5 mm for a 18F delivery system) [18].

Iliofemoral tortuosity does not predict vascular complications, but it can determine vascular elongation. In the case of severe tortuosity, the use of a stiff wire can be helpful, but particular attention should be paid to the distance between the access site and the aortic annulus [21].

For TF procedures, both percutaneous and cutdown access can be used: when the site of access is adequately large and without significant calcifications, percutaneous access is the first choice. In this case, the access is usually closed with various percutaneous devices available in commerce [11]. In the percutaneous approach, the anatomy of femoral artery should be always accurately studied, paying attention to the level of femoral bifurcation [19].

When the risk of percutaneous access is too high, it is preferable to opt for a cutdown approach, avoiding vascular complications in the site of puncture.

Several retrospective studies and one randomized trial have analyzed the differences in outcomes between a percutaneous approach and a surgical cutdown access. None of the available studies could demonstrate a superiority of a percutaneous approach, and the benefit of this choice remains controversial [22–24].

A step-by-step approach is mandatory in order to minimize the risk of complications.

General anesthesia is optional for transfemoral TAVI, but less used rather than the initial TAVI era.

The first step is to identify the femoral puncture site, ideally 1 cm above the femoral bifurcation. Usually, on the basis of CT scan, the best femoral access (right or left) is chosen. Two sheaths (6 Fr) are placed in the contralateral femoral artery and vein, so that a pigtail arterial catheter and a right ventricular pacemaker lead are placed [25].

To proceed more safely, in the case of percutaneous access, the puncture could be done under ultrasound view or fluoroscopy (preferably after a selective angiography from the contralateral site). A standard 0.035 inch wire is retrogradely introduced in the iliac-femoral axis, and a 8 Fr vascular introducer sheath is placed in order to predilate the artery before the placement of a preclosure suture devices. At this point, a 8 Fr sheath is reintroduced over a standard 0.035 guidewire, an Amplatz catheter is placed in descending aorta, and the previous guidewire is changed with a 260 cm stiff wire.

The native aortic valve is crossed by a straight tip guidewire with the support of an Amplatz catheter (AL1–AL2). Once the aortic valve is crossed, the catheter is replaced by a stiff wire with a pigtail curve, paying attention to the risk of ventricular perforation [26].

At this point, a balloon aortic valvuloplasty (BAV) could be performed. BAV is particularly useful in some settings: in very severe and calcified aortic valves, in the case of borderline transcatheter aortic valve sizes, in bicuspid aortic valves, and in the presence of very low coronary ostia to observe the movement of the aortic valvular leaflets.

Then, the transcatheter aortic bioprosthesis is advanced up to the aortic valve, being careful during aortic arch crossing.

The balloon-expandable prostheses need rapid ventricular pacing (180–200 bpm) during the deployment while for self-expanding valves are not mandatory.

It is important to find an optimal implantation plane. Usually, it is calculated before the procedure on the basis of CT scan and verified by angiography, in order to have a single plane with all three cusps aligned.

Once the valve has been implanted, it is necessary to evaluate, by angiography and echocardiography, the position of prosthesis (not too high or too low), the possible presence of perivalvular regurgitation, and the trans-prosthesis gradients.

To have an easier vascular access closure, in some centers, a crossover with a secure wire from the contralateral femoral artery is performed: in this way, a rapid balloon occlusion and/or a delivery of a covered stent could be performed. A final angiography should be performed to check the result.

3.4.2 Transapical TAVI

The transapical (TA) approach, first described by Ye and colleagues in 2006 [27], is historically considered the alternative to transfemoral access. Usually, it is performed when the peripheral axis is impractical. The presence of large apical thrombus represents the major contraindication to this procedure.

The apex can be localized by fluoroscopy, TTE, or TEE. The more appropriate site of puncture is on the LV apex, which is, usually, more anterior and proximal than anatomic cardiac apex [3].

For ventricular pacing, both intracavitary (via femoral vein) and epicardial ventricular leads could be positioned.

The apex is exposed via an anterolateral left anterior mini-thoracotomy in the fifth or sixth intercostal space, under general anesthesia. After placing two purse-string sutures at the puncture site, ventricular puncture is done, and a standard 0.035 inch guidewire is advanced across the degenerated aortic valve, paying attention to avoid mitral valve apparatus. After, with a support of a Judkins catheter, a long stiff wire (260 cm) is placed into the abdominal aorta. The delivery sheath is introduced into the ventricular cavity, and the balloon-expandable valve is opened during rapid ventricular pacing. The final result is checked by TOE and aortic ascending angiography.

The balloon-expandable valves (Edwards Sapien) are the most used in transapical access; anyway, self-expanding bioprostheses (Symetics or Jena-Valve) could be implanted having CE mark. In the latter case, there is no need for rapid ventricular pacing.

Possible complications of the TA approach are bleeding at the site of the apical puncture, myocardial tears, apical scarring, aneurysm formation, or chronic pain [28].

3.4.3 Alternative routes

For transaortic access, an upper partial sternotomy or a right mini-thoracotomy at the second or the third intercostal space can be performed. Felt-reinforced purse-string suture is placed in the ascending aorta 4–5 cm above the aortic valve. Once the aortic valve is crossed retrogradely with a guidewire, the procedure is similar to transapical approach [3]. There are few contraindications to transaortic access: chest deformities, porcelain aorta, very short ascending aorta, and previous CABG with patent grafts [18].

The left subclavian artery can be used as an alternative access; the proximal third of the axillary artery represents the ideal site. In the evaluation of the axillary access, the same principles for the TF approach should be kept in mind. Particular attention should be paid at the level of the emergency of left subclavian artery, because of high rate of localization of atherosclerotic calcific plaques. Most of the times, the surgical approach is preferred in case of choice of the trans-axillary access [18]. Most of the time, in the trans-axillary access, self-expanding prostheses are preferred over balloon-expandable.

Rarely, if all types of approaches are not adequate, the **trans-carotid** access could be a valid alternative.

4. Valve choice

Currently, the types of valves most implanted are balloon-expandable and self-expanding valves.

Basically, the choice of valve depends on anatomical considerations and available valve sizes. Attention should be paid to annulus dimension and its geometry, bicuspid/tricuspid valve, amount and distribution of calcifications in LVOT and proximal aorta, sino-tubular and ascending aorta dimensions, and coronary height [11].

Usually, in the case of extensive calcifications with an increased risk of rupture, in extreme oval-shape annulus or in the presence of iliofemoral diameter between 5.0 and 5.5 mm, a self-expanding valve is preferred [29–31].

Instead, when we are in the presence of dilated ascending aorta (> 43 mm), very angulated aorta (particularly for transfemoral approach), or in the presence of an elevated preoperative risk of postprocedural pacemaker implant, the choice can fall on the balloon-expandable valves.

Anyway, most of the time the choice depends on operator experience and confidence [3].

5. Conclusions

The use of TAVI in patients affected by aortic stenosis is spreading more and more, treating intermediate- and low-risk patients.

The selection of patients seems to be a crucial point, pointing out the role of the Heart Team.

MDCT is the technique of choice in preoperative planning: it provides information regarding aortic valve and vascular access. Particular attention should be paid on bicuspid valve morphology.

The choice of valve is, basically, based on confidence and experience of the operator and the center.

Author details

Antonio Giovanni Cammardella[1*], Federico Ranocchi[1], Antonio Lio[1], Amedeo Pergolini[1], Francesco Nicolò[1], Marina Comisso[1], Vitaliano Buffa[2] and Francesco Musumeci[1]

1 Department of Cardiac Surgery and Heart Transplantation, San Camillo Forlanini Hospital, Rome, Italy

2 Cardio-Vascular Radiology Unit, San Camillo Forlanini Hospital, Rome, Italy

*Address all correspondence to: agcammardella@gmail.com

References

[1] Durko AP, Osnabrugge RL, Van Mieghem NM, Milojevic M, Mylotte D, Nkomo VT, et al. Annual number of candidates for transcatheter aortic valve implantation per country: Current estimates and future projections. European Heart Journal. 2018;**39**(28):2635-2642

[2] De Sciscio P, Brubert J, De Sciscio M, Serrani M, Stasiak J, Moggridge GD. Quantifying the shift toward transcatheter aortic valve replacement in low-risk patients: A meta-analysis. Circulation. Cardiovascular Quality and Outcomes. 2017;**10**(6):e003287

[3] Otto CM, Kumbhani DJ, Alexander KP, Calhoon JH, Desai MY, Kaul S, et al. ACC expert consensus decision pathway for transcatheter aortic valve replacement in the management of adults with aortic stenosis: A report of the American College of Cardiology task force on clinical expert consensus documents. The Journal of the American College of Cardiology. 2017;**69**(10):1313-1346

[4] Baumgartner H, Falk V, Bax JJ, De Bonis M, Hamm C, Holm PJ, et al. ESC/EACTS guidelines for the management of valvular heart disease. The European Heart Journal. 2017;**38**(36):2739-2791

[5] Nishimura RA, Otto CM, Bonow RO, Carabello BA, Erwin JP 3rd, Fleisher LA, et al. 2017 AHA/ACC focused update of the 2014 AHA/ACC guideline for the management of patients with valvular heart disease: A report of the American College of Cardiology/American Heart Association task force on clinical practice guidelines. Circulation. 2017;**135**(25):e1159-e1e95

[6] Bax JJ, Delgado V, Bapat V, Baumgartner H, Collet JP, Erbel R, et al. Open issues in transcatheter aortic valve implantation. Part 1: Patient selection and treatment strategy for transcatheter aortic valve implantation. European Heart Journal. 2014;**35**(38):2627-2638

[7] Blanke P et al. Computed tomography imaging in the context of transcatheter aortic valve implantation (TAVI)/Transcatheter aortic valve replacement (TAVR): An expert consensus document of the Society of Cardiovascular Computed Tomography. JACC: Cardiovascular Imaging. 2019;**12**(1):1-24

[8] Roberts WC, Janning KG, Ko JM, Filardo G, Matter GJ. Frequency of congenitally bicuspid aortic valves in patients >/=80 years of age undergoing aortic valve replacement for aortic stenosis (with or without aortic regurgitation) and implications for transcatheter aortic valve implantation. The American Journal of Cardiology. 2012;**109**(11):1632-1636

[9] Mack MJ, Brennan JM, Brindis R, Carroll J, Edwards F, Grover F, et al. Outcomes following transcatheter aortic valve replacement in the United States. Journal of the American Medical Association. 2013;**310**(19):2069-2077

[10] Sievers HH, Schmidtke C. A classification system for the bicuspid aortic valve from 304 surgical specimens. The Journal of Thoracic and Cardiovascular Surgery. 2007;**133**(5):1226-1233

[11] Jilaihawi H, Chen M, Webb J, Himbert D, Ruiz CE, Rodes-Cabau J, et al. A bicuspid aortic valve imaging classification for the TAVR era. JACC: Cardiovascular Imaging. 2016;**9**(10):1145-1158

[12] Yoon S-H, Bleiziffer S, De Backer O, et al. Outcomes in transcatheter aortic valve replacement for bicuspid versus tricuspid aortic valve stenosis. Journal

of the American College of Cardiology. 2017;**69**(21):2579-2589

[13] Abdel-Wahab M, Zahn R, Horack M, Gerckens U, Schuler G, Sievert H, et al. Transcatheter aortic valve implantation in patients with and without concomitant coronary artery disease: Comparison of characteristics and early outcome in the German multicenter TAVI registry. Clinical Research in Cardiology. 2012;**101**(12):973-981

[14] Leon MB, Smith CR, Mack MJ, Makkar RR, Svensson LG, Kodali SK, et al. Transcatheter or surgical aortic-valve replacement in intermediate-risk patients. The New England Journal of Medicine. 2016;**374**(17):1609-1620

[15] Reardon MJ, Van Mieghem NM, Popma JJ, Kleiman NS, Sondergaard L, Mumtaz M, et al. Surgical or transcatheter aortic-valve replacement in intermediate-risk patients. The New England Journal of Medicine. 2017;**376**(14):1321-1331

[16] Kotronias RA, Kwok CS, George S, Capodanno D, Ludman PF, Townend JN, et al. Transcatheter aortic valve implantation with or without percutaneous coronary artery revascularization strategy: A systematic review and meta-analysis. Journal of the American Heart Association. 2017;**6**(6)

[17] Bax JJ, Delgado V, Bapat V, Baumgartner H, Collet JP, Erbel R, et al. Open issues in transcatheter aortic valve implantation. Part 2: Procedural issues and outcomes after transcatheter aortic valve implantation. European Heart Journal. 2014;**35**(38):2639-2654

[18] Biasco L, Ferrari E, Pedrazzini G, Faletra F, Moccetti T, Petracca F, et al. Access sites for TAVI: Patient selection criteria, technical aspects, and outcomes. Frontiers in Cardiovascular Medicine. 2018;**5**:88

[19] Blanke P, Weir-McCall JR, Achenbach S, Delgado V, Hausleiter J, Jilaihawi H, et al. Computed tomography imaging in the context of transcatheter aortic valve implantation (TAVI)/transcatheter aortic valve replacement (TAVR): An expert consensus document of the society of cardiovascular computed tomography. JACC Cardiovasc Imaging. 2019;**12**(1):1-24

[20] Okuyama K, Jilaihawi H, Kashif M, Takahashi N, Chakravarty T, Pokhrel H, et al. Transfemoral access assessment for transcatheter aortic valve replacement: Evidence-based application of computed tomography over invasive angiography. Circulation. Cardiovascular Imaging. 2015;**8**(1)

[21] Toggweiler S, Gurvitch R, Leipsic J, Wood DA, Willson AB, Binder RK, et al. Percutaneous aortic valve replacement: Vascular outcomes with a fully percutaneous procedure. Journal of the American College of Cardiology. 2012;**59**(2):113-118

[22] Genereux P, Webb JG, Svensson LG, Kodali SK, Satler LF, Fearon WF, et al. Vascular complications after transcatheter aortic valve replacement: Insights from the PARTNER (placement of AoRTic TraNscathetER valve) trial. Journal of the American College of Cardiology. 2012;**60**(12):1043-1052

[23] Kadakia MB, Herrmann HC, Desai ND, Fox Z, Ogbara J, Anwaruddin S, et al. Factors associated with vascular complications in patients undergoing balloon-expandable transfemoral transcatheter aortic valve replacement via open versus percutaneous approaches. Circulation. Cardiovascular Interventions. 2014;**7**(4):570-576

[24] Bernardi FL, Gomes WF, de Brito FS Jr, Mangione JA, Sarmento-Leite R, Siqueira D, et al. Surgical cutdown

versus percutaneous access in transfemoral transcatheter aortic valve implantation: Insights from the Brazilian TAVI registry. Catheterization and Cardiovascular Interventions. 2015;**86**(3):501-505

[25] Cribier A, Litzler PY, Eltchaninoff H, Godin M, Tron C, Bauer F, et al. Technique of transcatheter aortic valve implantation with the Edwards-Sapien heart valve using the transfemoral approach. Herz. 2009;**34**(5):347-356

[26] Stortecky S, Buellesfeld L, Wenaweser P, Windecker S. Transcatheter aortic valve implantation: The procedure. Heart. 2012;**98**(Suppl 4): iv44-iv51

[27] Ye J, Cheung A, Lichtenstein SV, Carere RG, Thompson CR, Pasupati S, et al. Transapical aortic valve implantation in humans. The Journal of Thoracic and Cardiovascular Surgery. 2006;**131**(5):1194-1196

[28] Pascual I, Carro A, Avanzas P, Hernandez-Vaquero D, Diaz R, Rozado J, et al. Vascular approaches for transcatheter aortic valve implantation. Journal of Thoracic Disease. 2017;**9**(Suppl 6):S478-SS87

[29] Koehler T, Buege M, Schleiting H, Seyfarth M, Tiroch K, Vorpahl M. Changes of the eSheath outer dimensions used for transfemoral transcatheter aortic valve replacement. BioMed Research International. 2015;**2015**:572681

[30] Kasel AM, Cassese S, Bleiziffer S, Amaki M, Hahn RT, Kastrati A, et al. Standardized imaging for aortic annular sizing: Implications for transcatheter valve selection. JACC: Cardiovascular Imaging. 2013;**6**(2):249-262

[31] Hansson NC, Norgaard BL, Barbanti M, Nielsen NE, Yang TH, Tamburino C, et al. The impact of calcium volume and distribution in aortic root injury related to balloon-expandable transcatheter aortic valve replacement. Journal of Cardiovascular Computed Tomography. 2015;**9**(5):382-392